Avoiding the Medicaid Trap

Avoiding the Medicaid Trap

How to Beat the

Catastrophic Costs of

Nursing-Home Care

Armond D. Budish

A DONALD HUTTER BOOK

HENRY HOLT AND COMPANY   NEW YORK

To my loving family: Amy, Ryan, Daniel, Janice, Irving, and Doris

"... let us hope that the heritage of old age is not despair."

Benjamin Disraeli
(*Vivian Grey* [1826],
Book VIII, Chapter 4)

Published by Henry Holt and Company, Inc.,
115 West 18th Street, New York, New York 10011.
Published in Canada by Fitzhenry & Whiteside Limited,
195 Allstate Parkway, Markham, Ontario L3R 4T8.

LIBRARY OF CONGRESS CATALOGING-IN-PUBLICATION DATA
Budish, Armond D.
Avoiding the Medicaid trap : how to beat the catastrophic
costs of nursing-home care / Armond D. Budish.—1st ed.
    p. cm.
"A Donald Hutter book."
ISBN 0-8050-1035-1
1. Nursing-home care—United States—Costs. 2. Medicaid.
3. Financial security.   I. Title.
RA997.B795   1989
338.4'33621'60973—dc19   88-34617
                                                  CIP

Henry Holt books are available at special discounts
for bulk purchases for sales promotions, premiums,
fund-raising, or educational use. Special editions
or book excerpts can also be created to specification.

For details contact:
Special Sales Director
Henry Holt and Company, Inc.
115 West 18th Street
New York, New York 10011

Designed by Beth Tondreau Design
Printed in the United States of America
10 9 8 7 6 5

The Durable General Power of Attorney form on
pages 93–95 is reprinted with permission from the June 1,
1987, issue of *Family Circle* magazine. Copyright © 1987
The Family Circle, Inc.

Contents

Introduction

The toughest decision you may ever have to make is to place your parent or spouse into a nursing home. No one ever wants to take that step. But there may come a time when there's just no choice—an older person may develop Alzheimer's disease, crippling arthritis, or some other severely debilitating condition that requires full-time care and attention, which you, the offspring or spouse, can't offer.

More than a million times a year, Americans find that their options have run out and their only alternative is to admit a loved one to a nursing home.

The decision to institutionalize a parent or spouse raises many tough questions. Are you abandoning your loved one when he or she needs you most? How will he or she react to being moved from a familiar home environment to an impersonal facility? Will your parent or spouse receive adequate medical care? How will the staff treat him or her? Although many nursing homes offer excellent services, we've all heard horror stories too.

While issues like these create extreme emotional trauma, that trauma often pales in comparison with the *financial* shock of having to pay for long-term nursing care. Claude M. Pepper, U.S. representative from Florida and the leading advocate for senior citizens' rights in our country today, has recognized: "The single greatest fear of our senior citizens, and of all Americans [is] that a long-term catastrophic illness may strike and, because of the absence of public or private coverage, they will become destitute."[1]

With nursing-home bills of $2,000/month ($24,000/year) or *more*, that fear is well founded. A million Americans *every year* are forced into destitution, which means they have had to give up their home and their savings to pay their bills from a catastrophic illness.

Jack Ossofsky, president of the National Council on Aging, described exactly the kind of devastating impact a long-term illness can have within just a few weeks or months of a loved one's entry into a nursing home:

> For an older couple of average income, a diagnosis of Alzheimer's disease spells the impoverishment of the well partner within 4 months, as the couple is forced to spend down to meet medicaid assets and income requirements for nursing home care. . . . [W]e are forcing Americans to impoverish themselves to get minimal coverage for the needs they face.[2]

These statistics have very real faces behind them—they represent people who were not acting irresponsibly, people who did the best they could although it wasn't enough. Listen to the story of Grace Still:

> In 1982, [my mother] was diagnosed with Alzheimer's disease.
>
> Although Dad was disabled himself, he wanted to take care of Mom. He did for several years. . . .
>
> Mom was a strain for him to handle even with an aide to help him. Every time we could provide the care ourselves in our home we did. But both my sister and I are single parents working full-time jobs.

It broke our hearts but Mom became too much for all of us to handle, and we had to place her in a nursing home.

The tragedy of Mom's stay in the nursing home is the cost. Most of their life savings, almost $30,000, is gone now. The home care and companion services for Mom and Dad amounted to $280 a week, costing $1700 for only six weeks. *Dad has paid $15,000 in only six months for the nursing home care which costs approximately $2200 a month.* Mom is receiving medical assistance now. *All she has left is a fund for her burial.*

My Dad worked hard as a machine operator for thirty years. He always took good care of Mom, my sister and me, and provided us with a good living. He had insurance from Blue Cross and Blue Shield in addition to his Medicare. It is heartbreaking for him to see her receiving welfare because his life savings have been wiped out, and his own health is failing. . . .

It is a disgrace to our great nation that our elderly must be absolutely destitute or dying before they can receive help.

Mom and Dad have been struggling with their illnesses for ten years. Because their ailments are incurable or chronic diseases, no health insurance will cover their custodial expenses. Their only crime is that they worked hard not to be a burden all these years, only to have everything they had taken out from under them.[3]

After placing his wife of forty-nine years in a nursing home, Nathan Mendelsohn was faced with a similar crisis:

After Rose had a stroke in 1982, it became evident that our life savings and health insurance policies were not going to be enough to cover the expenses. After rehabilitation and therapy for several weeks, Rose was left partially paralyzed.

For months, I cared for her myself, keeping the house, dressing and bathing her, and then carrying her downstairs for the day. But I am 77 years old and I am not as strong as I used to be. Caring for Rose at home in our two-story house got to be too much of a strain for me. . . .

Medicare coverage and all other insurance coverage stopped. I began paying $2300 a month for the nursing home. In six months' time, I spent $20,700 for her nursing home care.

Besides paying for the nursing home, I had to pay my rent, and had to pay for food, gas and electricity each month. . . .

I have little left from the money that we gained from the sale of our home. I am 77 years old. If something should happen to me, I don't know what I would do. I do not want to be a burden to my family.[4]

Nursing-home patients and their families often are stripped of everything: their homes, their savings, their dreams. Spouses of nursing-home patients may be left destitute and even forced onto the welfare rolls. And then what incentive is left for nursing-home patients, whether married or unmarried, to try to get better and return home—to homes they no longer own and to daily living expenses they can no longer afford? Why is this permitted to happen?

U.S. Representative Robert A. Borski of Pennsylvania asked the right question: "Why should our citizens bankrupt themselves, become dependent on the state and be robbed of their dignity and self-esteem because they suffer from 'uncovered' or chronic illnesses?" Why indeed! Borski goes on: "What is most disheartening is that . . . the financial devastation is unnecessary."[5]

Yes, the financial devastation *is* unnecessary. You don't have to sit by idly while a financial nightmare becomes reality. *The tips in this book can save you and your family thousands of dollars!* By planning ahead, or assisting your parents or spouse to plan ahead, you can help maintain a loved one's dignity and preserve family savings from being completely lost to a nursing home.

Successful planning means having to address facts that many of us don't feel comfortable discussing. If you have older parents, they, like most older people, probably like to believe that they'll always be independent. Nobody wants to think he or she will be struck down by a catastrophic illness or injury that requires long-term care. And when you consider that, of all persons entering nursing homes, over 80 percent are not married at the time, you can see why children often must bear the burden of assisting a parent to prepare a suitable Medicaid plan and to gain admittance to a nursing home.

If planning can be so helpful, why don't we hear more about ways older Americans can protect assets? Why doesn't the government promote planning?

The answer is simple—it would cost Uncle Sam a lot of money.

In fact, government bureaucrats will even go out

of their way to *prevent* you from finding out how to protect yourself and your family. Here is an example of the type of resistance I have encountered when trying to explain the options available to our senior citizens.

In a lengthy Letter to the Editor of the *Cleveland Plain Dealer*, Paul Offner, Medicaid director for the state of Ohio, responded to an article I wrote promoting Medicaid planning by stating:

> Medicaid is the government program of health care for the poor. It was created so that those who had no other way of paying their health bills could still obtain medical care. But that's not Budish's view. "Juggle your assets," he tells his readers, so that you too can become Medicaid-eligible, whether you're poor or not. If you are elderly and are contemplating nursing home care, transfer your assets to a relative or a friend so that, at least on paper, you'll look poor. That way you can "conserve your savings" while having the taxpayer pick up the nursing home bill.
>
> Unfortunately, there are numerous lawyers like Budish running around, and there are more people following his advice. The result, eventually, will be that legislatures will have to find some way to penalize this willful divestiture of assets to become Medicaid-eligible. I hope your readers will turn their backs on those who would turn us all into an army of cynics playing the loopholes and seeking the unethical shortcuts in life.

Offner goes on to state that Medicaid planning is "reprehensible" and those who do so are "selfish."

If trying to help your parents or spouse avoid losing their life savings is "selfish," so be it. But it's *not* reprehensible. What is reprehensible is that politicians and Medicaid bureaucrats, like Mr. Offner, have shut their eyes to this colossal problem and are allowing families to be devastated by nursing-home costs.

As you can see, Offner doesn't question the efficacy of the planning techniques offered in this book. He just attacks me as being immoral because I am trying to help people "take advantage" of the present system.

Not everyone believes that it is "reprehensible" to try to help one's parents or spouse protect their life savings. Congressman Claude Pepper, chairman of the Subcommittee on Health and Long-Term Care, Select Committee on Aging, expressed his "enthusiastic support" for this book:

> The advice in this book is crucial to older Americans, to help them protect their savings and avoid impoverishment. I am enthusiastic in supporting this publication which presents important information not to my knowledge found anywhere else.

Unfortunately, there is only one Claude Pepper—few other politicians are willing to stand up for older Americans.

Even liberal U.S. Representative Pete Stark of California has referred to instances of planning as "cheating cases where parents deed houses to kids and apply for Medicaid."

Is it immoral, as Medicaid bureaucrats and politicians suggest, to consider ways to avoid poverty? Absolutely not!

Isn't it far more immoral that our government forces its citizens to deplete their life savings on nursing homes? The goal of sound public policy should be to prevent this sort of financial devastation. As stated by noted attorneys Michael Gilfix and Peter J. Strauss in their article "New Age Estate Planning: The Emergence of Elder Law" (*Trusts & Estates Magazine*, April 1988): "Reasonable asset preservation has been at the top of the national legislative agenda for years; it is not the creature of creative, scurrilous lawyers trying to find that illicit edge for his or her client."

In fact, haven't Americans for years been allowed to take advantage of tax protections and deductions to preseve their assets from taxes—without criticism from the politicians? What's the real difference between middle-class Americans using tax deductions to protect assets from Uncle Sam and the elderly using trusts to protect some assets from the nursing home? Why criticize the elderly? As Gilfix and Strauss so aptly stated:

> [P]lanning to preserve a portion of one's estate when facing long-term care is conceptually tantamount to arranging one's personal finances to take maximum advantage of tax protections and deductions. In both circumstances the attorney advises the client about opportunities presented by law and regulations to minimize the loss of assets. Tax planning and tax advice are and have been "mainstream" for decades. Asset preservation planning in the face of long-term care is not yet mainstream, but is rapidly emerging.

Isn't it amazing that here in the United States our politicians would have us believe that planning for our family's financial survival is immoral? It's not planning that's immoral; it's our government policies. These policies force our elderly to leave everything—money, property, pride, and dignity—on the steps of the nursing home as they enter.

Other Western countries have adopted far more humane systems than we have in the United States. For example, the Canadian government guarantees its citizens long-term nursing-home care *without* requiring residents to impoverish themselves and their families.

A variety of proposals to fund long-term care for middle-income Americans has been made. Many senior citizen advocate groups have urged funding by taxes, maybe "sin" taxes on alcohol and tobacco, to spread the burden of costs from families with members in nursing homes to the general population. Others have suggested developing a system in which private insurance would cover the first year or two and the government would pay the nursing-home expenses after that.

Most Americans are willing to pay their fair share for nursing-home costs. But in this country, that is not an option. Older Americans and their families are *forced* into poverty to pay nursing-home costs unless they take steps to protect themselves. Unfortunately, few people plan ahead.

Consumer advocate Esther Peterson, who herself is eighty-two, hit the nail on the head when she said:

> We've done very poor planning. When you get up into your older years, you don't want to be a burden. You want to be independent and want to protect whatever resources you have. We have been so slow in waking up to this.[6]

It's time to wake up and start planning. Perhaps someday we will see the adoption of a humane government policy on nursing-home financing, and then every older American will be able to get whatever care is best for him or her without being financially, as well as emotionally, devastated. But until then, the financial burden rests with the family.

The tips in this book are intended primarily to benefit middle-income Americans. As U.S. Senator John Heinz of Pennsylvania has stated: "The greatest threat to the financial security of middle-income Americans is the cost of long-term medical care."[7] Those persons with very little income and assets probably are adequately protected by existing law; the Medicaid rules were designed specifically to help the poor. The wealthy can and should pay their fair share. But if you are one of the great majority of Americans falling in between, this book can save you and/or your family thousands of dollars.

1 | What, Me Worry About Nursing-Home Costs?

The statistics are horrifying: elderly persons aged sixty-five to sixty-nine years face almost a *one-in-two risk of entering a nursing home!*[1]

Surprised by such a high risk? You shouldn't be. As Esther Peterson, a consumer-movement pioneer and longtime advocate for the elderly, points out, a wide variety of illnesses and injuries could land a loved one in a nursing home:

> Most people think of catastrophic illness as a massive heart attack, a bone-crushing auto accident, or cancer. But the biggest catastrophe of all well may be the crippling, chronic conditions—such as senility, Alzheimer's disease, severe arthritis, osteoporosis, or the long-term effects of a stroke.[2]

Our older population is the fastest-growing segment in the country. Right now, well over 30 million Americans are sixty-five and older, and 7 million of them need long-term care. Government statistics show the number of people over age eighty—those most in need of long-term care—to be over 6 million now and doubling by 2010. Within the next fifty years, more than one in five citizens, about 60 million strong, will be elderly, and many of them, more than 19 million, will need long-term care.

There now are 2.3 million elderly in nursing homes; in thirty years, almost *double* that number will wind up institutionalized. By 1988 alone, Blue Cross and Blue Shield estimates 1.2 million elderly will be admitted to nursing homes.

A poll conducted for the American Association of Retired Persons (AARP) and the Villers Foundation determined that long-term care and its costs already touch many of us. Sixty percent of respondents in the poll had some personal experience, through family or friends, with long-term care. More than half of the respondents expected that, within the next five years, someone in their own families would require long-term care.

Congresswoman Mary Rose Oakar of Ohio highlighted the same views in congressional hearings:

> All of us can recite at least one incidence when a loved one or close friend has needed extended assistance at no fault of their own. Perhaps it is one of our parents, perhaps one of our children or a neighbor. It is normally a situation of great misfortune where the health of the individual is suddenly swept away to expose the fact that our lives are precarious and in need of constant care. How many of us now have a parent or a close friend facing not only the frustrations of poor health but also financial ruin due to an extended illness or injury? Almost every one can relate at least one occurrence of such a tragedy. This is not the problem of an isolated few.[3]

Of course, all this probably comes as no great surprise. In all likelihood, you too know someone whose life has been traumatized by the financial strains brought on by illness and long-term care.

The High Costs of Nursing-Home Care

The costs of nursing-home care are soaring and are already far beyond the means of most of us. The average cost of nursing-home care is about $2,000/month, or $24,000/year. And that's if you're lucky. In many metropolitan areas like New York City, nursing homes charge as much as $50,000 to $75,000 annually. And even if nursing homes around you are charging "only" $24,000, don't breathe a sigh of relief yet; in thirty years, the *average* annual costs are expected to more than double to $55,000.

The average nursing-home stay is more than two years, but many elderly citizens will spend far more time than that in a "golden age home."

Consider Alzheimer's disease, which has struck more than 7 percent of the nation's elderly over age sixty-five. Although victims must often be placed in a nursing home, Alzheimer's disease does not necessarily reduce a person's life expectancy. A patient with Alzheimer's lives an average of *eight years* after the symptoms first appear, with much of that time often spent in a nursing home.

Long-term illnesses like Alzheimer's disease are emotionally devastating; with care costs at $2,000/month, these illnesses can financially wipe out a family.

How Nursing-Home Costs Devastate a Family

Here's how it all adds up:

> High Nursing-Home Costs + Lengthy Stays = Disaster for Your Family

Anyone who has had a family member or friend enter a nursing home knows only too well the accuracy of this formula.

California Congressman Edward R. Roybal, chairman of the House Select Committee on Aging, put this formula into words:

> Millions of elderly and non-elderly Americans are at great personal financial risk of being impoverished by high and sustained long term care costs. With over 200 million Americans underinsured against long term care costs . . . , *a host of personal catastrophes are in the making.*[4]

How long will your family be able to hold out? How long will it take to dissipate the nest egg your parents or spouse worked so hard during their lifetimes to build up? The sad answer is: Not long.

By using Tables 1 and 2, you can estimate how long your (as an older person) or your parents' financial resources would last. For example, if your mother is living alone, has income of between $6,000 and $10,000 and average assets for that income range, the nursing home would get everything after she spent just *32 weeks* in the facility. If she were to be "fortunate" enough to recover so that she could leave the nursing home and return to the community after that time, she would be facing life on the welfare rolls! These figures in Tables 1 and 2 explain why elderly Americans and their families fear not only the health impact of a long-term illness, but also the financial devastation that often follows.

The devastation of a nursing-home stay has already wrecked the lives of countless older Americans and their families. Let a few people tell you, in their own words, about the pending disaster if a family member suffers a catastrophic health problem and needs full-time care:

Mrs. Bellamy

> I'm writing to tell you about my husband. My son had to put him in a nursing home today. He has had two strokes. I've waited on him, and me sick. See I live by a pacemaker and can hardly walk because of arthritis. The doctor said I could no longer care for him because I couldn't lift him or give a bath or give him IV's. So he had to go to a nursing home.
>
> We are both 74 years old and I feel God has been good to us both. He worked until he was 70 years and paid into Social Security ever since 1937. He sure wasn't lazy.
>
> Now, all of our life savings are gone. Henry and I together got $831 in Social Security. Today the nursing home will take $562 of his, and that will leave me $269 to live on, which sure will be rough going, even with the sickness I have.[5]

Placing a loved one in a nursing home is a draining experience—both emotionally and financially:

Mary H. Housel

> My husband was ill for 10 years prior to his death. I was able to maintain his care at home for 7½ years. . . . When I could not manage his care at home any longer, I was able to place him in a nursing home where he remained for 2½ years before he died. The cost of nursing home care, medicines and doctors' care depleted our life savings.[6]

Our government's lack of commitment to long-term-care assistance has forced many Americans and their families into a terrible situation with no good options for relief.

Samuel L. Baily
> My mother died of Huntington's Disease [a hereditary, terminal brain disorder that results in the gradual loss of control over both the body and the mind]. . . . I am at risk for HD and I have a wife and three children whom I love and for whom I wish to provide as best I can. We are not wealthy, but we do have some savings and a house. I believe I should pay my fair share, but I do not believe I should be forced to strip my family of these assets if I should get HD. My options at present are to divorce my wife or to commit suicide neither of which I intend to do.[7]

These are not unique cases. The ruination brought upon the elderly and their families by unbearable nursing-home costs is widespread, touching virtually every American in all walks of life.

Representative Pepper, in a hearing before his House Select Committee on Aging, Subcommittee on Health and Long-Term Care, recognized that these stories "could be matched in every city in America and in every part of this nation. People have suffered similarly to these people. . . . Every one of them lost their homes. Every one of them lost their savings. And every one of them suffered terribly in America."[8]

The House Select Committee on Aging recently produced a report entitled "Long Term Care and Personal Impoverishment: Seven in Ten Elderly Living Alone Are at Risk." The results of that report were astounding: *seven in ten elderly living alone find their income depleted to the federal poverty level after only thirteen weeks in a nursing home.* This means that, after about three months, 70 percent of unmarried older Americans have insufficient income to pay their monthly nursing-home bills. After the same thirteen weeks, nearly one-half of the elderly living alone have used up both their income and their financial assets. Within one year, two-thirds of older Americans living alone have lost everything.

Married couples' financial resources don't last

TABLE 1

Average Number of Weeks to Poverty for Unmarried Older Americans in Nursing Homes

AVERAGE ASSETS AND ANNUAL INCOME	NO. OF WEEKS TO POVERTY IF AGE 65	NO. OF WEEKS TO POVERTY IF AGE 75
$4,860–$6,075	8	9
$6,075–$9,720	32	36
$9,720–$15,000	97	110

SOURCE: Select Committee on Aging, U.S. House of Representatives, October 1987.

TABLE 2

Average Number of Weeks to Poverty for Married Older Americans with One Spouse in a Nursing Home

AVERAGE ASSETS AND ANNUAL INCOME	NO. OF WEEKS TO POVERTY IF AGE 65	NO. OF WEEKS TO POVERTY IF AGE 75
$6,540–$8,175	18	21
$8,175–$13,000	27	32
$13,000–$20,000	94	108

SOURCE: Select Committee on Aging, U.S. House of Representatives, October 1987.

much longer after one spouse enters a nursing home. Over one-half of all elderly couples see their income dissipate down to the poverty line after one spouse has spent just six months in a nursing home. *After twelve months, nearly one-half of all couples with one spouse in a nursing home have lost their entire nest egg.*

As Tables 3 and 4 clearly demonstrate, it's just a matter of time—and not much time—until a loved one will be forced into poverty after entering a nursing home. By planning ahead and following the steps described in the next few chapters, you, your spouse, and/or your parents can protect yourselves and your family.

TABLE 3

Risk of Impoverishment for Unmarried Americans in Nursing Homes

NO. OF WEEKS IN NURSING HOME	PERCENTAGE OF SINGLE ELDERLY WHO BECOME IMPOVERISHED	
	Based on Income and Assets	*Based on Income Alone*
13	48%	69%
26	58%	84%
39	63%	91%
52	67%	94%

SOURCE: Select Committee on Aging, U.S. House of Representatives, October 1987.

TABLE 4

Risk of Impoverishment for Elderly Couples with One Spouse in a Nursing Home

NO. OF WEEKS IN NURSING HOME	PERCENTAGE OF ELDERLY COUPLES WHO BECOME IMPOVERISHED	
	Based on Income and Assets	*Based on Income Alone*
13	22%	34%
26	34%	56%
39	41%	69%
52	46%	78%

SOURCE: Select Committee on Aging, U.S. House of Representatives, October 1987.

2 | Who Pays the Bill?

Total nursing-home costs in our country are expected to be $46 billion in 1988. In thirty years, they are expected to be $100 billion. If a person must enter a nursing home, part of these costs will be billed to him or her.

You may never have worried about nursing-home costs because you've always assumed someone else—maybe Medicare, maybe private insurance—would pick up the tab. Well, you and your family had better start to worry, because chances are that *no* person, *no* government program, and *no* insurance coverage will protect your family's savings from the grasp of a nursing home.

Representative Borski recognized:

> If you have the misfortune of getting a long-term catastrophic illness in the United States of America, no one will help you. Not the United States Government and Medicare, not Medigap insurance policies and no one until you have exhausted all of your financial resources, until they ask you to become virtually penniless, until you lose your home, until you lose all of your money, and unfortunately until you lose all of your pride.[1]

Nursing homes are businesses. When a loved one enters a nursing home, someone will have to pay the bill. Five sources for payment are most often considered:

- Medicare
- Private insurance
- Veterans' Administration benefits
- Medicaid
- Personal assets and savings

Relying solely on the last option can be ruinous. It doesn't take a trained mathematician to figure out the impact on a person's savings if he or she has to foot the entire bill. Ideally, if government or private insurance lent a hand, the odds that you and your family could manage would be increased.

The reality is that none of these other sources is much help, leaving most older Americans at risk of losing everything to a nursing home.

Medicare

Medicare is widely available, covering more than 30 million Americans. It is federal health insurance for all persons over age sixty-five who are entitled to monthly Social Security or Railroad Retirement benefits. Even persons under sixty-five are eligible if they have received Social Security disability benefits for two years.

With so many people protected by Medicare, why is long-term nursing care such a problem? Won't Medicare cover the costs of long-term care?

Let's explode that dangerous myth right now— *neither Medicare nor private insurance will pay for nursing-home costs!* It can't be said any more clearly. Don't count on Medicare to pay for a nursing home.

Of all those receiving Medicare benefits, only one-tenth of 1 percent are covered for nursing-home care. Yet people believe otherwise: An AARP survey indicated that 80 percent of Medicare beneficiaries believed they were adequately protected from the high costs of long-term care by Medicare and their private policies. In fact, Medicare pays less than 2 percent of the nation's long-term nursing-care bill. Why do so few qualify? The answer is simple: Medicare coverage is extremely limited. It provides only limited coverage of home health and skilled nursing care—when a person is suffering an acute illness and needs rehabilitation or therapy to recover—and no coverage for custodial care.

At *most*, Medicare will pay 80 percent of nursing-home costs for eight days and all the costs for up to 142 more days. Any stay longer than 150 days and your family is on its own. (For all the hoopla, the Medicare Catastrophic Coverage Act added only fifty days to covered nursing-home stays.) Since statistics show that an older person is likely to remain in a nursing home for two years or more, Medicare isn't going to solve the cost problem.

It's tough to qualify for even this limited 150-day Medicare coverage. To have Medicare pay *any* nursing-home costs:

- The care a person receives must be "medically necessary," which means skilled care, not intermediate or custodial care.
- The nursing home must be a Medicare-approved skilled nursing facility with a registered nurse available seven days a week, twenty-four hours a day.
- The bed the person is assigned must be Medicare-certified.
- As a practical matter, the person can receive the necessary care only at a nursing home providing *skilled* care.

These tests are rarely satisfied. Skilled care generally includes medical or therapeutic services that can be performed only by or under the supervision of nurses, physical therapists, or other medically trained professionals. For example, if a doctor or nurse observes a patient's condition, develops a plan of treatment and/or care, prescribes medications, inserts a catheter, administers injections, applies surgical dressings, treats skin problems, or provides physical or speech therapy, the care should qualify as "skilled" care.

Skilled care is very different from custodial care, which is much more typically required for long periods. Custodial care helps people dress, bathe, eat, take medication, and carry on other normal living activities. It can be provided by individuals with no special medical training. If a loved one is stricken with Alzheimer's disease, Parkinson's disease, senility, or a stroke, he or she may need custodial care—not skilled care—for a long time, yet Medicare won't cover the costs.

Besides skilled nursing-home care, there are other options available to older people for long-term needs, options that may or may not be covered by Medicare. They include:

Home Health Care. Just as it sounds, it provides health care services at home. Services range from skilled nursing care and speech, physical, and occupational therapy to homemaker or companion services. Even small home repairs and yard work may be included.

Medicare provides limited coverage (e.g., visits by a skilled nurse-practitioner of up to five days a week for twenty-one days, then up to six days a week for thirty-eight days beginning in 1990) only if the need is certified by a doctor, if the care includes part-time or full-time skilled nursing care, physical therapy, or speech therapy, and if the agency providing the home care participates in Medicare. Otherwise, your parent or spouse is on his or her own.

Hospice Care. Provided for the terminally ill, hospice care is designed to ease one's suffering, not to cure or rehabilitate. Hospice care can be provided at home or in a hospice facility. Either way, the costs are high, but Medicare covers a substantial portion. (The Medicare Catastrophic Coverage Act of 1988 eliminated the ceiling of 210 days of coverage.)

Adult Day Care. Provides company for, or supervision to, people at home who need just companionship or minimal assistance during the day. Costs generally are not covered by Medicare or Medicaid.

Respite Care. Very short-term health or custodial care provided at home or in a nursing home in order to give family members who normally care for the individual a rest. The patient will probably have to pay most or all of these costs. Beginning in 1990, the Medicare Catastrophic Coverage Act provides coverage for up to eighty hours a year of professional care for a homebound patient, to relieve an unpaid family member or friend.

Meals on Wheels. Provides hot meals at home periodically. Costs are not covered by Medicare or Medicaid, but they may be part of some other federal or state government program.

Forget Medicare as an answer to long-term nursing-care needs. If you (or a loved one) can qualify for Medicare at all—and chances of that are slim—at most you will get some help toward your bills for 150 days. If you initially qualify for Medicare by meeting all the requirements, and then care is reduced to custodial care, you will lose Medicare coverage even if the 150-day period hasn't yet expired. On average, Medicare covers less than two weeks of a person's nursing-home stay. After 150 days, you will be on your own no matter what.

Private Insurance

Private insurance is even less helpful than Medicare, covering only about 1 percent of all nursing-home costs. Again, many older Americans have been sadly misled into believing that their so-called Medigap or Medifil supplemental insurance policies will pay for any necessary long-term care. Here is a typical story:

Jack J. Lomas

> My aunt . . . is confined to a nursing home, stripped of all her worldly earnings. . . .
>
> My aunt worked from the time she was fourteen, for over fifty years, in a textile mill, toiling long hours for very little money. In the process, she lost her hearing and her health. She has cataracts, colitis and a chronic heart condition, in addition to arthritis in her legs and spine and other chronic health problems. The country she worked so hard to support in her youth and vigor has turned its back on her during her time of need.
>
> She purchased Blue Cross–65 Special and a supplemental insurance policy from AARP to pick up what Medicare did not pay. She thought she was well taken care of. But when she went into the nursing home, her life savings, almost $13,000, were eaten up in just six months. Medicare, Blue Cross–65 Special and AARP will not cover the expenses because the care she needs is called custodial. Because she suffers from chronic illness, none of the insurers will pay for her medical care to keep her comfortable.[2]

Representative Robert A. Borski stated at a recent congressional hearing:

> Older Americans unknowingly pay exorbitant prices for policies which do not provide relief from the high medical costs associated with chronic illnesses. . . . Clearly, the private insurers are not picking up the tab for extended nursing care.[3]

Representative Claude Pepper shared that view:

> Senior citizens buy hope in the form of one or more insurance policies, not realizing that there is no public or private insurance policy, or combination of such policies, that will protect them when a catastrophic illness strikes and provide them with the comprehensive coverage they desperately want.[4]

Is there truly "no public or private insurance policy" that covers long-term care in a nursing home? Just about. Fewer than 500,000 persons in the entire country have policies that actually cover long-term nursing-home care.

Why are so many of our nation's elderly fooled into believing that supplemental private Medigap insurance policies cover long-term care? Stanley J. Brody, professor of health care systems at the Wharton School of the University of Pennsylvania and director of the Research and Training Center for Rehabilitation of Elderly Disabled Individuals, correctly put his finger on the cause when he said that "media marketing methods by private insurers . . . lull elderly consumers into believing they are covered for long-term care." In other words, many in the Medigap insurance industry have intentionally set out to deceive older Americans in order to make a buck.

In fact, many insurers haven't been satisfied to sell one worthless policy to a consumer; some have been known to use scare tactics and high-pressure techniques to sell several overlapping policies to a single person.

Esther Peterson warned: "High-power salesmen have talked people into thinking they need things. I talked to one woman who had seven policies. Only one of them was worth anything." One woman from Arkansas was duped into buying twenty-eight Medigap policies, none of which paid her a single penny toward her nursing-home charges.

Gail Shearer, manager in charge of policy analysis for Consumers Union (publisher of *Consumer Reports*), also had few kind words for private long-term insurance providers. According to Ms. Shearer, private policies are marketed to the elderly "often through deceptive marketing techniques." As a result, Consumers Union initiated litigation in California to try to "halt the unfair and deceptive marketing of Medigap insurance to senior citizens."[5] Shearer said that, as a result of confusion, "older Americans waste $3 billion annually on private health insurance."[6]

About seventy private insurers actually offer long-term-care coverage. Those few policies that do offer nursing-home-care coverage are, in the words of the House Select Committee on Aging, "woefully inadequate for protecting lower and middle income Americans." The reason: the premiums are often too high and the benefits typically too limited for most Americans. In particular:

- Annual premiums range from $300 to a whopping $15,000, depending on the insured's age and the options chosen.
- Benefit payments are restricted.
- Scope of coverage is limited.
- Certain diseases, such as Alzheimer's, are often excluded.
- Qualification requirements are tough to satisfy.

Val J. Halamandaris, president of the National Association for Home Care, gave very poor marks to private long-term-care insurance on the market:

There is no product on the market worthy of the name long-term care insurance, at least nothing I would recommend to anyone. The policies that exist are riddled with exceptions such as prior hospitalization requirements, they are not indexed to inflation and they, with one exception, fail to provide meaningful home care coverage. . . . [To provide real protection], the premium would have to be set at levels well beyond what people could afford to pay.[7]

The pros and cons of long-term-care insurance are discussed in Chapter 10. Suffice it to say now that private insurance probably isn't the answer to the nursing-home cost dilemma.

Veterans' Administration Benefits

If an older person is a veteran, he or she may be entitled to limited nursing-home coverage. VA benefits are available only if:

- The patient was in a VA hospital and is being directly discharged into a nursing home. Or:

- The patient's need for a nursing home stems from a service-connected disability, which is defined as an injury or disease incurred or aggravated in the line of duty.

Even if you or a loved one should qualify, don't expect much. VA benefits generally won't last for any more than six months.

Medicaid

Medicaid *will* cover long-term care in a nursing home; in fact, about 40 percent of our nation's nursing-home costs are paid by Uncle Sam and the states through the Medicaid program. Medicaid has become the largest payer—by far—for long-term care.

But there's a hitch, and it's a *huge* one. To qualify for Medicaid, a person must either be poor or become poor. As one person testified before a congressional committee, the "law is without pity" when it comes to government financing for nursing-home costs:

Loving Child in Cicero, Illinois
> Pop had to be put in a nursing home at a cost to my mother of about $2,400 per month, and neither Medicare nor Medicaid could help because my parents had a nest egg. The law is without pity. Had my father lived for just 2 more years in a nursing home, my mother would have had to spend the rest of her life in poverty, but God called Pop to his eternal rest in 1 year, rather than 2. My mother and I can never forget the terrible feeling of relief we had when Pop died. We can only live with it in shame. We loved him.[8]

Medicaid bureaucrats like to say that lower- and middle-income Americans must "spend down" their resources before Medicaid coverage begins. That's a nice euphemism—"spend down." In plain English it means that a person must turn over his or her life savings to the nursing home before Medicaid will pay a cent.

The House Select Committee on Aging accurately described the picture:

> Medicaid coverage comes with a heavy price for persons needing long term care as well as their spouses. . . . [T]he bottom line is that elderly persons must essentially impoverish themselves, and probably their spouses, before they are protected by Medicaid.[9]

Say your parents are not poor before one of them enters a nursing home. With nursing-home costs as high as they are, your parents will surely become poor before long. According to the U.S. Department of Health and Human Services, about one-half of the people receiving Medicaid coverage for nursing-home costs had too much money or property to qualify when they first entered but became impoverished—and so qualified for Medicaid—after entering the home.

How many people are losing their life savings to nursing homes? The figures represent a terrible human tragedy and national embarrassment. More than *500,000 people each and every year* qualify for Medicaid help in paying nursing-home expenses by exhausting their own resources.

So Medicaid will help pay nursing-home costs, but at the price of financial ruin.

Personal Assets and Savings

If you or your parents end up paying for the nursing home, you or they will pay until money runs out.

About one-half of all long-term care is paid by elderly Americans and their families. In 1984 (the latest federal statistics), this came to $13 billion— a lot of money by any measure.

Most older citizens have annual incomes of $11,554 or less. When you compare this figure with average annual nursing-home costs of $24,000, you can see that older Americans have got a real problem.

If a person starts early in life, can he or she save enough to avoid impoverishment? That would be the ideal solution. Unfortunately, it's not very realistic. Let's say your father put $1,000 each year into an interest-bearing account beginning when he was forty. Twenty-five years later, he wouldn't have saved enough to pay for even a year and a half in a nursing home!

As you can see, a family's life savings is at serious risk when a loved one enters a nursing home. Uncle Sam and insurance carriers aren't likely to be much help. You and your parents will have to take action to avoid financial tragedy.

3 How Much Can an Older Person Keep from the Nursing Home?

For most older people, the general rule is simple: Anything you have (your income and life savings) must go to the nursing home to pay expenses. Only when your assets run out will Medicaid step in.

As shown in the preceding chapter, this rule has a devastating impact on older Americans and their families. Already the system has failed millions of older Americans. Congress recently tried to remedy the situation by including some protections in the Medicare Catastrophic Coverage Act of 1988. That legislation was designed to keep the spouse remaining at home (called the "spouse-at-home" or the "community spouse") from impoverishment when a mate entered a nursing home.

Unfortunately, the great promise of the Medicare Catastrophic Coverage Act remains largely unfulfilled. The act will have no impact on the costs of long-term nursing care for most older Americans: It is directed solely at married couples with one spouse in a nursing home. Yet fewer than one in five nursing-home residents are married at the time of their admission, and that number dwindles over time. For most older Americans with no spouse at home, the law remains as it was—completely "without pity."

For married couples, the Medicare Catastrophic Coverage Act may *harm* as many people as it helps with respect to financing nursing-home care. The law allows the spouse-at-home to avoid total destitution but removes some of the best and easiest planning options that previously allowed older citizens to protect a portion of their assets. Although the new law makes it a little harder, older people can still take steps to protect their finances.

This book will not burden you with all the details of the Medicaid qualification rules as they now stand. But it is important to understand some of them, so as to better plan to protect the family nest egg from the ravages of nursing-home costs.

To qualify for Medicaid, a person entering a nursing home must:

- Be at least sixty-five, blind, or disabled (as defined by the state).
- Need the type of care provided in a nursing home (more than thirty states have preadmission screening programs).
- Meet the income limitation test.
- Meet the assets limitation test.

So long as the person meets these criteria, Medicaid generally will cover long-term nursing-home care.

Below is a brief description of the Medicaid income and assets limitation tests. Since different rules apply to married and nonmarried people, we'll look at each group separately.

Nonmarried Individuals

INCOME LIMITATION TEST

Eligibility Standards

In most states, there is no limit on the amount of income you may have in order to qualify for Medicaid. In these states, listed in Table 5, you meet

TABLE 5

States with No Limit on Income for Older Individuals Seeking Medicaid Coverage for Nursing-Home Costs

California	Nebraska
Connecticut	New Hampshire
District of Columbia	New York
Hawaii	North Carolina
Illinois	North Dakota
Indiana	Ohio
Kansas	Oregon
Kentucky	Pennsylvania
Maine	Rhode Island
Maryland	Utah
Massachusetts	Vermont
Michigan	Virginia
Minnesota	Washington
Missouri	West Virginia
Montana	Wisconsin

SOURCE: Edward Neuschler, *Medicaid Eligibility for the Elderly in Need of Long Term Care* (Report Prepared under Contract for the Congressional Research Service). Washington, D.C.: National Governors' Association Center for Policy Research (hereafter "National Governors' Association Report"). Tables from the National Governors' Association Report generally reflect the most recent information effective as of July 1, 1987. Although most of the information remains accurate today (or has been updated), readers are advised to check with their state for exact information.

TABLE 6

States with a $1,062 Limit* on Monthly Income for Older Americans Seeking Medicaid Coverage for Nursing-Home Bills

Alaska	New Jersey
Arkansas	Oklahoma
Colorado	South Carolina
Florida	South Dakota
Idaho	Tennessee
Iowa	Wyoming
Louisiana	

*The $1,062 income limit refers to total income from all sources before any deductions for 1988; the 1989 figure was not available at this writing but will be slightly higher.

SOURCE: National Governors' Association Report.

TABLE 7

States with Monthly Income Limits* Below $1,062 for Older Americans Seeking Medicaid Coverage for Nursing-Home Bills

STATE	INCOME LIMIT
Alabama	$852.90
Delaware	632.00
Georgia	937.00 (Net)
Nevada	734.00
New Mexico	871.00
Texas	658.65

*The income limits refer to total income from all sources before any deductions, unless otherwise indicated. Net income refers to income after application of any disregards and deductions applied to determine Medicaid eligibility (normally the first $20 of unearned income is disregarded). In Florida and Georgia, in addition to the net income limit, gross income cannot exceed $1,062.

SOURCE: National Governors' Association Report.

the eligibility standards whether your income is $20/month or $2,000/month.

Even if you don't live in one of the twenty-nine states (and the District of Columbia) with no income limits, you still stand a good chance of passing the income limitation test, unless your income is fairly high. In the thirteen states listed in Table 6, you can meet the eligibility standards with an income up to $1,062/month. The remaining six states listed in Table 7 use lower income limits.

What do these income figures mean? They mean that, for most people, the income limitation test will be no problem. According to the most recent census data, the majority of older Americans have incomes well below these limits. (The median monthly income in 1985 for men sixty-five and older was $908, and for women sixty-five and older it was $526; only 45 percent of elderly men and 21 percent of elderly women had incomes above these figures.) In other words, qualifying for Medicaid should not pose a problem for most older Americans *who can also pass the tougher assets limitation test.*

How Much Income Can an Older Person Keep?

Say your widowed or divorced mother is eligible under the income limitation test. In that event, almost all of her income must go to the nursing home. Only if her income (and assets) isn't enough to pay the whole bill will Medicaid step in.

She can protect a small amount of her income. In particular, she will get:

- A monthly allowance for her personal, non-medical needs, such as clothing, toiletries, books, and magazines, from $30 to $70, depending on the state. The specific amounts allowed are listed in Table 8.

- In most states, credit toward her nursing-home bill for any funds spent for health insurance premiums, including Medicare premiums, and other medical expenses not covered by Medicaid, such as glasses, dentures, hearing aids, and over-the-counter drugs. (Federal law actually requires *all* states to provide this credit, but not all of them do.)
- In just over one-half the states, an allowance to help her maintain her home in anticipation of returning within three to six months after entering a nursing home. As Table 9 shows, in most states she could keep about $200/month, with figures ranging from $75 to over $600/month. Generally, this home-maintenance allowance is available only for unmarried individuals and only upon a physician's statement that he or she should be able to return to the

home within six months; if a nursing-home stay exceeds six months, this allowance normally cuts off after that time.

Here's an example of how these rules work:

Example 1

Your mother lives in New York and enters Sunny Hills nursing home. The doctor assures her she'll be able to return home within a few months. Her monthly income is $1,000. She may keep:

$40	for her personal-needs allowance (from Table 8)
$65	for her medical insurance premium
$417	for her home-maintenance allowance (from Table 9)
Total $522	a month

The nursing home would get the rest of her income, $478/month.

TABLE 8

Personal-Needs Allowance Protected Out of Individual Income

STATE	AMOUNT	STATE	AMOUNT
Alabama	$30	Montana	$40
Alaska	70	Nebraska	30
Arkansas	30	Nevada	35
California	35	New Hampshire	35
Colorado	30	New Jersey	35
Connecticut	40	New Mexico	30
Delaware	31	New York	40
District of Columbia	60	North Carolina	30
Florida	30	North Dakota	45
Georgia	30	Ohio	30
Hawaii	30	Oklahoma	30
Idaho	30	Oregon	30
Illinois	30	Pennsylvania	30
Indiana	30	Rhode Island	30
Iowa	30	South Carolina	30
Kansas	30	South Dakota	30
Kentucky	40	Tennessee	30
Louisiana	33	Texas	30
Maine	35	Utah	30
Maryland	40	Vermont	40
Massachusetts	65	Virginia	30
Michigan	32	Washington	36.62
Minnesota	40	West Virginia	30
Mississippi	44	Wisconsin	40
Missouri	30	Wyoming	30

SOURCE: National Governors' Association Report.

TABLE 9

States Providing a Home-Maintenance Allowance

STATE	AMOUNT*	FLAT OR MAXIMUM† AMOUNT	MAXIMUM NO. OF MONTHS AVAILABLE
Alaska	$632	Flat	6
California	192	Flat	6
Colorado	185	Flat	6
Connecticut	Varies	Maximum	3
Delaware	75	Flat	None
District of Columbia	391	Flat	None
Idaho	212	Flat	6
Illinois	Varies	Maximum	6
Maryland	334	Flat	6
Massachusetts	455	Maximum	6
Minnesota	402	Maximum	3
Montana	340	Flat	6
Nebraska	140	Flat	6
New Hampshire	141	Flat	3
New Jersey	150	Maximum	6
New York	417	Flat	6 Subject to extension
North Carolina	242	Flat	6
North Dakota	345	Flat	6
Oregon	Varies	None	None
Pennsylvania	372.40	Flat	6
Rhode Island	491.67	Maximum	6
South Carolina	340	Flat	6
Utah	262	Flat	6
Vermont	299	Flat	6
Virginia	Varies	Maximum	6
Washington	180	Flat	6
West Virginia	175	Flat	None
Wisconsin	442.72	Flat	6
Wyoming	150	Flat	6

*In the second column, "Varies" indicates that a home-maintenance allowance is provided, but that the amounts vary according to a state formula.
†In the third column, "Flat" indicates that this amount in all cases is the home-maintenance allowance; "Maximum" indicates the most that will be permitted under a formula adopted by the state.

SOURCE: National Governors' Association Report.

To qualify for Medicaid, a person must pass the income limitation test. That generally means that one's income must be less than the nursing-home costs—an easy test to pass for most older Americans. Once you qualify, you will be able to keep only a small portion of your income and the rest will go to pay the bills.

ASSETS LIMITATION TEST

As if it weren't bad enough that, under the income limitation test, most of an older person's income will go to a nursing home, the assets limitation test is worse: under that test, almost all of a person's assets also must be turned over to the nursing home before Medicaid will pay a penny of the nursing-home charges. If one is not poor going into the nursing home, it won't take long to get there.

For purposes of the assets limitation test, an older person's assets include almost all of his or her money and property. Most states define assets as "cash or other liquid assets or any real or personal property that an individual (or spouse, if any) owns and could convert to cash." Say your father has to pass the

18

test. His assets will include his cash, savings and checking accounts, CDs, stocks, bonds, mutual fund shares, promissory notes, cars, and real estate.

Now, I don't want to overstate the case. Our elected officials, in their generosity, will allow an older person to keep some of his or her assets up to a maximum total value of about $2,000 (plus certain exempt assets), depending on which state he or she lives in. Just think, your parent works a lifetime, and for all that sweat he or she will get to keep a grand sum of $2,000. Table 10 lists the amount of assets each state allows a person to protect from a nursing home.

In addition to about $2,000, a few specific items (called exempt assets) are excluded from the maximum asset allotments listed in Table 10. Although these protected assets vary from state to state, the most common include:

- A person's home. This is protected as long as a spouse or a dependent relative is living there. And even if no dependent relative or spouse is living there, the home may still be protected—most states will allow the house to remain protected as long as its owner intends to return there; in some states, the house will remain protected only for a limited time. Table 11 shows the rules adopted in each state for protecting a home.
- Household goods and other personal items up to a total (equity) value of $2,000.
- One wedding ring and one engagement ring, regardless of value.
- One car (or other vehicle) with a current market value of up to $4,500. No limit on value if the car is necessary to get to work or to receive medical care, or if the car has been adapted for a handicapped person.

TABLE 10

**Amount of Assets a Person Can Protect
from a Nursing Home**

STATE	AMOUNT	STATE	AMOUNT
Alabama	$2,000	Montana	$2,000
Alaska	2,000	Nebraska	1,600
Arkansas	2,000	Nevada	2,000
California	2,000	New Hampshire	2,500
Colorado	2,000	New Jersey	2,000
Connecticut	1,600	New Mexico	2,000
Delaware	2,000	New York	3,000
District of Columbia	2,600	North Carolina	1,500
Florida	2,000	North Dakota	3,000
Georgia	2,000	Ohio	1,500
Hawaii	2,000	Oklahoma	2,000
Idaho	2,000	Oregon	2,000
Illinois	2,000	Pennsylvania	2,400
Indiana	1,500	Rhode Island	4,000
Iowa	2,000	South Carolina	2,000
Kansas	2,000	South Dakota	2,000
Kentucky	2,000	Tennessee	2,000
Louisiana	2,000	Texas	2,000
Maine	2,000	Utah	2,000
Maryland	2,500	Vermont	2,000
Massachusetts	2,000	Virginia	2,000
Michigan	2,000	Washington	2,000
Minnesota	3,750	West Virginia	2,000
Mississippi	2,000	Wisconsin	2,000
Missouri	999.99	Wyoming	2,000

SOURCE: National Governors' Association Report.

TABLE 11

Rules for Protecting a Person's House from a Nursing Home[a]

STATE	YOU WILL BE PROTECTED:			ANY TIME LIMIT ON PROTECTION?
	If You Intend to Return[b]	*If Your Doctor Certifies That You Are Likely to Recover Enough to Return*	*Whether or Not You Return*	
Alabama[c]	X			No
Alaska	X	X		No
Arkansas	X			No
California	X			No
Colorado	X			No
Connecticut[c]		X		9 mos.
Delaware	X			No
District of Columbia	X			No
Florida	X			No
Georgia	X			No
Hawaii	X			No
Idaho	X			No
Illinois	X			No
Indiana[d]	X			No
Iowa	X			No
Kansas[e]	X			No
Kentucky			X	No
Louisiana	X			No
Maine	X			No
Maryland[c]	X			No
Massachusetts			X	No
Michigan			X	No
Minnesota			X	6 mos.
Mississippi	X			No
Missouri[f]			X	No
Montana		X		6 mos.
Nebraska		X		6 mos.
Nevada		X		No
New Hampshire[e]		X		No
New Jersey		X		6 mos.
New Mexico	X	X		No
New York		X		No
North Carolina		X		6 mos.

(continued on next page)

- Up to $6,000 equity in property (personal and real estate) if essential to the person's support. To be considered necessary for support, the property should either produce income or produce goods or services necessary for one's daily activities (such as land to grow food for one's own use). Income-producing property should produce net annual income of at least 6 percent of the amount of protected equity.
- Cash surrender value of life insurance *if* the total face value of all life insurance on any one person doesn't exceed $1,500.

- Burial plots for the person and his or her immediate family.
- Up to $1,500/person for burial costs if kept separate from other resources.

All but fourteen states have adopted the asset protection rules (other than for a home) described above. Table 12 lists the most significant variations adopted by the fourteen remaining states.

People often are confused about the protection available for equity in property essential to an older

TABLE 11 (continued)

Rules for Protecting a Person's House from a Nursing Home[a]

STATE	YOU WILL BE PROTECTED:			ANY TIME LIMIT ON PROTECTION?
	If You Intend to Return[b]	If Your Doctor Certifies That You Are Likely to Recover Enough to Return	Whether or Not You Return	
North Dakota		X		6 mos.
Ohio			X	6 mos.
Oklahoma	X	X		12 mos.
Oregon		X		6 mos.
Pennsylvania	X			No
Rhode Island	X			No
South Carolina	X			No
South Dakota	X	X		6 mos.
Tennessee	X			No
Texas	X			No
Utah	X			No
Vermont	X			No
Virginia		X		6 mos.
Washington	X			No
West Virginia	X			No
Wisconsin		X		6 mos.
Wyoming	X			No

[a]This table assumes that the older person has no spouse or dependent relative at home. If he or she does, the house is protected.

[b]The statement that you intend to return home must usually be made in writing.

[c]States have been permitted to adopt lien laws, allowing them to place liens on the homes of nursing-home residents receiving Medicaid. Liens may not be placed on a home if living there is the nursing-home resident's spouse, dependent children, or sibling who has an ownership interest in the home and has been living there for a year. A nursing-home resident can probably block the imposition of a lien just by stating in writing his or her intent to return home. In any event, only three states, Alabama, Connecticut, and Maryland, have adopted lien laws to date.

[d]For residents of Indiana, one's home will be protected until either one has no intent to return or one is physically unable to return.

[e]For residents of Kansas, a home will be protected for three months without regard to whether the person will return; for residents of New Hampshire, a home will be protected for six months without regard to whether the person will return.

[f]For residents of Missouri, the state has a $23,000 limit on total assets, including the equity in one's house, until October 1, 1989. So if a person owns a home worth more than $23,000 (or less with other assets), he or she will have to sell the home and turn at least part of the proceeds over to the nursing home. After October 1, 1989, one's home becomes a completely protected asset regardless of its value.

SOURCE: National Governors' Association Report.

person's support. Here's an example to illustrate that exclusion.

Example 2

Your mother has a small business in her house making handwoven rugs. The looms and other equipment used in the business have a value of $7,000, and her equity is $5,500 since she owes $1,500 on the looms. Your mother's income (net of expenses) is $400. Since her equity in the looms and other equipment ($5,500) is under the $6,000 limit for property essential to her support, and since her net income ($400) is greater than 6 percent of her equity, your mother's looms and other equipment would be excluded from the maximum asset allotments listed in Table 12.

The assets limitation test can and usually does have a devastating impact on nursing-home residents and their families. It requires residents to spend virtually their entire life savings on a nursing home before Medicaid helps, *unless* they take steps to prepare.

Married Individuals

The new Medicare Catastrophic Coverage Act throws a few crumbs to a nursing-home resident's spouse-at-home. Unfortunately, the meat and potatoes still go to the nursing home.

INCOME LIMITATION TEST

Eligibility Standards

In general, the eligibility standards for someone who is married are the same as for an unmarried individual—if one's income is below the amounts set forth in Tables 5, 6, and 7, the person should pass the income eligibility test.

But let's say your husband is entering a nursing home. How much of his and your total joint income will be considered to be his and how much will be considered yours? How is income to be divided between spouses?

Just about every state has answered these questions by assuming that income belongs to the spouse whose name is on the check, unless there's some reason to say otherwise. (Hence it is called the "name-on-the-check" rule.) Money paid to your husband from his pension or Social Security is considered to be his; income paid to you is considered to be yours—even if the two of you use the incomes jointly.

In two states—California and Washington—the rule is a little different. These two states apply community-property rules, which generally means that you and your spouse each are considered to own one-half of any income, regardless of whose name is on the check. Yet even these two states apply their community-property rules instead of the general "name-on-the-check" rule only when it benefits the spouse-at-home and use the "name-on-the-check" rule when *that* is better for the spouse-at-home.

Although only California and Washington now apply community-property rules to determine income for Medicaid-eligibility purposes, other community-property states may adopt similar rules in the future. Table 13 lists such states; if you or your parents live in one of these states, check to see which rules that state now uses for determining income for Medicaid-eligibility purposes.

After dividing the income between spouses, three states require another adjustment before deciding whether the nursing-home resident's income is under or over the eligibility limit. Indiana, Nebraska, and West Virginia will "add" some of the income from the spouse-at-home to the income of the spouse in the nursing home (the "nursing-home spouse"):

Indiana: Any income of a spouse-at-home over $674/month is "added" to the nursing-home spouse's income unless it can be shown that his or her actual living expenses exceed $674.

Nebraska: Any income of a spouse-at-home over $391/month (after certain deductions) is "added" to the nursing-home spouse's income.

West Virginia: Any income of a spouse-at-home over $200/month (after certain deductions) is "added" to the nursing-home spouse's income.

If a nursing-home spouse lives in one of the remaining forty-seven states, no income from his or her spouse-at-home is counted in the other's income (starting with the month after the nursing-home spouse entered the nursing home) when deciding on one's income eligibility for Medicaid.

How Much Can a Nursing-Home Spouse Keep?

Once you have determined that your nursing-home spouse is *eligible* for Medicaid under the income test, put aside your calculations and start again to find out exactly how much of his or her income can be kept. Beginning September 30, 1989, these rules are much different from the eligibility rules.

Again, use the "name-on-the-check" rule to allocate income between you and your spouse. If income is paid in your spouse's name, it will be considered his or hers; income paid in your name is considered yours. Income paid jointly to both of you is considered to be shared equally. If others, such as children or business partners, are named on the income payment, the income is considered as a *pro rata* payment to each named person. Payments received from a trust are considered in the same way as income from any other source, *unless* the trust says otherwise. This will be important when it comes to planning for a nursing-home spouse.

In years past, this method of income allocation often left a spouse-at-home with no income. Let's say your father worked his entire life, building up his pension and Social Security, which now provide him a nice stream of income. While your father was working outside the home, your mother may have taken care of the unpaid chores, raising the children and maintaining the house, *not* earning a pension. If your father had gone into the nursing home, his

TABLE 12

Assets Excluded from Medicaid Asset Eligibility Limits (Other Than Home)

STATE	HOUSEHOLD GOODS	RINGS	CAR	INCOME-PRODUCING PROPERTY	OTHER PROPERTY FOR SUPPORT	LIFE INSURANCE	BURIAL PLOTS	BURIAL COSTS
Connecticut	Up to $2,000	1 wedding, 1 engagement	1 up to $4,500	No equity limit	No limit	Excluded if face value below $1,500	Excluded	Excluded up to $1,100
Hawaii	No jewelry except rings; all other household goods, no limit on value	1 wedding, 1 engagement	1 up to $1,500				Excluded	Excluded up to $1,500
Illinois	Up to $2,000	1 wedding, 1 engagement	All vehicles fully exempt unless primarily for recreation	No equity limit	No limit	Excluded if face value below $1,500	Excluded	Excluded up to $1,500
Indiana	No limit	1 wedding, 1 engagement	1 up to $4,500	Excluded up to $6,000, if property produces 6% return on excluded equity	Real property excluded only if producing food for home consumption	Excluded if face value below $1,400 and policy beneficiary is recipient's estate or funeral director	Excluded	Excluded only if irrevocable
Minnesota	No limit	1 wedding, 1 engagement	1 up to $500	Excluded up to $6,000, if property produces 6% return on excluded equity	Not excluded unless not salable	Excluded if face value below $1,500	Excluded	Excluded up to $1,500
Missouri	No limit	1 wedding, 1 engagement	1 vehicle without limit on value	No equity limit if used in trade or business		Excluded if face value below $1,500	Excluded	Excluded only if irrevocable
Nebraska	Household goods of "moderate value"	1 wedding, 1 engagement	1 up to $1,500			Excluded if face value below $1,500	Excluded	Excluded only if irrevocable

State								
New Hampshire	No limit	1 wedding, 1 engagement	All vehicles fully exempt	No equity limit, excluded as long as income exceeds expenses		Excluded if face value below $1,500	Excluded	Excluded only if irrevocable or for persons who are medically needy*
North Carolina	No limit	1 wedding, 1 engagement	1 up to $4,500	Excluded up to $6,000, if property produces 6% return on excluded equity		Excluded if face value below $1,500—maximum for couple	Excluded	Excluded up to $1,500
North Dakota	Up to $2,000	1 wedding, 1 engagement	1 up to $4,500	Excluded up to $6,000, if property produces 6% return on excluded equity	Equity up to $6,000 excluded	Excluded if face value below $1,500	Excluded	Excluded up to $1,500
Ohio	No limit	1 wedding, 1 engagement	1 up to $4,500	Excluded up to $6,000, but if equity exceeds $6,000, entire equity is counted		Excluded if face value below $1,500	Excluded	Excluded only if irrevocable
Oklahoma	No limit	1 wedding, 1 engagement	1 up to $4,500	Excluded up to $6,000, if property produces 6% return on excluded equity	Equity up to $6,000 excluded	Excluded if face value below $1,500	Excluded	Excluded up to $1,500
Utah	Up to $2,000	1 wedding, 1 engagement	1 up to $4,500	Excluded up to $6,000, if property produces 6% return on excluded equity	Equity up to $6,000 excluded	Excluded if face value below $1,500	Excluded	Excluded up to $1,500
Virginia	No limit	1 wedding, 1 engagement	1 vehicle without regard to purpose or value	Excluded up to $6,000, if property produces 6% return on excluded equity	Generally not excluded unless not salable	Excluded if face value below $1,500	Excluded	Excluded only if irrevocable

*The medically needy are those people who do not receive cash assistance (Supplemental Security Income or state supplement) but who have limited income and resources and need help paying their bills.

SOURCE: National Governors' Association Report.

TABLE 13

Community-Property States

Arizona
California
Idaho
Louisiana
Nevada
New Mexico
Texas
Washington

SOURCE: National Governors' Association Report.

stream of income would have flowed into the nursing home's coffers while your mother might have been left with no alternative but welfare!

Statistics show that it has been women who have suffered the most. Because women typically live longer and earn less, the wife at home has been the one who most often has become destitute.

In an attempt to deal with this problem, the Medicare Catastrophic Coverage Act provides a basic living allowance to support the spouse-at-home.

Spouse-at-Home Basic Living Allowance. The amount of the basic living allowance provided by Congress for the spouse-at-home is determined by a complicated formula. This should come as no surprise when you consider it was created by the same Congress that brought you the 1986 "tax simplification" law. To calculate the amount a nursing-home spouse can protect for his or her spouse-at-home:

1. Take 122 percent of one-twelfth of the income official poverty line for a family of two. At this writing, that would be $786/month.
2. For the principal residence of the spouse-at-home, add monthly rent or mortgage payments (including principal and interest); real estate taxes; homeowners' or renters' insurance costs; the state utility allowance or, if your state doesn't have one, actual average utility payments; and, for a condominium or cooperative, required maintenance charges (minus any included utility costs).
3. Take 30 percent of the amount in no. 1 above: today that is $235.80.
4. Calculate the amount by which the figure arrived at in no. 2 exceeds the figure in no. 3.
5. Take your figures from nos. 1 and 4 and add them together.

6. Subtract any income otherwise available to the spouse-at-home (income paid in his or her name plus one-half of joint income) from the amount in no. 5.

The amount in no. 6 gives you the basic living allowance that a nursing-home spouse can protect from his or her income for the spouse-at-home. (The 122 percent figure in no. 1 is effective starting September 30, 1989, and increases slightly in future years. In addition, the income official poverty line is adjusted periodically.)

Here are two examples of how this formula works:

Example 3

Your father's income is $2,000/month, and the income of his spouse who remains at home is $200/month. His spouse has rental and utility costs of $400/month.

1. 122 percent of one-twelfth of the poverty line is *$786/month.*
2. The residence costs for your father's spouse are *$400/month.*
3. 30 percent of the amount in no. 1 is *$235.80.*
4. No. 2 exceeds no. 3 by *$164.20* ($400 minus $235.80).
5. Nos. 1 and 4 together total *$950.20* ($786 plus $164.20).
6. Subtract $200 (the spouse-at-home's other income) from the amount in no. 5, and you get *$750.20.* So, of your father's income of $2,000/month, $750.20 would go to his spouse and $1,249.80 (less the personal-needs allowance and unreimbursed medical expenses, discussed next) would go to the nursing home.

Example 4

Your father's income is $3,000/month, and the income of his spouse who remains at home is $400/month. His spouse pays mortgage, utility, and insurance costs of $600/month.

1. 122 percent of one-twelfth of the poverty line is *$786.*
2. Your father's spouse pays residence costs of *$600.*
3. 30 percent of no. 1 is *$235.80.*
4. No. 2 exceeds no. 3 by *$364.20.*
5. Nos. 1 and 4 together total *$1,150.20.*
6. Subtracting his spouse's $400 income from the amount in no. 5, you get *$750.20.* So, of your

father's income of $3,000/month, $750.20 would go to his spouse and $2249.80 (less the personal-needs allowance and the unreimbursed medical expenses) would wind up paid to the nursing home.

Still, Congress wanted to make sure that a spouse-at-home didn't get *too* much money, so it put a $1,500/month cap on the basic living allowance for a spouse-at-home. (Note that some states may decide just to allow all spouses-at-home a flat $1,500 basic living allowance, without regard to the complicated formula. But no state has yet done so at the time of this writing.)

Following is a checklist to help calculate the basic living allowance.

SPOUSE-AT-HOME BASIC LIVING ALLOWANCE CHECKLIST

Instructions

Monthly Amount

1. 122 percent of one-twelfth of poverty line is: $786.00
2. (a) Monthly rent or mortgage payments (principal and interest) are: _____
   (b) Real estate taxes per month are: _____
   (c) Homeowners' or renters' insurance per month is: _____
   (d) Average utility costs per month are: _____
   (e) Condominium or cooperative maintenance charges (minus included utility costs) per month are: _____
   (f) Nos. 1 and 2(a)–(e) added together total: _____
3. 30 percent of amount in no. 1 is: $235.80
4. No. 2(f) minus no. 3 is: _____
5. No. 1 plus no. 4 is: _____
6. (a) Income of spouse-at-home is: _____
   (b) No. 5 minus no. 6(a), the basic living allowance, is: _____

By allowing a nursing-home spouse to give his or her spouse-at-home this basic living allowance, Congress has helped ensure that the spouse-at-home won't be left without any income, although as Examples 3 and 4 show, most of a nursing-home spouse's income is still likely to go to pay for long-term nursing care.

However, the basic living allowance will not help a spouse-at-home much, if at all, if the nursing-home spouse's income is close to or less than the income of the spouse-at-home. Looking at Example 3, if your father's and his spouse's monthly income was $1,100 each, *none* of your father's income could be paid to his spouse. In Example 4, if your father's monthly income was $2,200 and his spouse's monthly income was $1,200, *none* of your father's income could be paid to his spouse.

There are two important exceptions to the basic living allowance rules discussed above.

First, if a court has ordered a nursing-home spouse to pay a monthly amount to support his or her spouse-at-home, that takes precedence and would be the amount the nursing-home spouse would pay. At this time, very few states (with New York as the principal exception) have followed this approach. And support orders are no panacea anyway—even if a nursing-home spouse can use a support order to preserve more income for his or her spouse-at-home, the nursing-home spouse would have to hire a lawyer and go to court to get the order, a process that can be costly and time consuming (and often difficult for a nursing-home candidate or resident to manage).

Second, if the basic living allowance does not allow the spouse-at-home enough income, a higher amount may be permitted. However, exceptions are made only in *very rare circumstances* where it can be shown that the spouse-at-home will suffer *significant* financial duress unless more income is allowed.

Finally, note that the basic living allowance, like most provisions of the Medicare Catastrophic Coverage Act that relate to nursing homes, does not become available until September 30, 1989. Until that time, a spouse remaining at home is limited to a very small allowance ranging from $0 to $632/month, depending on which state he or she lives in. Table 14 indicates the maintenance allowances applicable until September 30. (Unless another date is stated, you can assume that September 30, 1989, is the effective date for provisions of the Medicare Catastrophic Coverage Act cited in this book.)

TABLE 14

**Maintenance-Needs Allowance Protected for a
Spouse-at-Home Through September 30, 1989**

STATE	PROTECTED DOLLAR AMOUNT	STATE	PROTECTED DOLLAR AMOUNT
Alabama	$354.00	Montana	$354.00
Alaska	632.00	Nebraska	375.00
Arkansas	187.80	Nevada	173.00
California[a]	550.00	New Hampshire	354.00
Colorado	229.00	New Jersey	371.25
Connecticut[b,c]	458.33	New Mexico	354.00
Delaware	354.00	New York[c,d]	417.00
District of Columbia	362.00	North Carolina	242.00
Florida	354.00	North Dakota	345.00
Georgia	354.00	Ohio[e]	258.00
Hawaii	300.00	Oklahoma	-0-
Idaho	413.00	Oregon	341.70
Illinois[b,c]	Varies	Pennsylvania	372.40
Indiana	354.00	Rhode Island	491.67
Iowa	354.00	South Carolina	354.00
Kansas	341.00	South Dakota	257.00
Kentucky	192.00	Tennessee	150.00
Louisiana	186.80	Texas	354.00
Maine	354.00	Utah	289.00
Maryland[c]	334.00	Vermont[b]	656.00
Massachusetts	455.00	Virginia[b]	325.00
Michigan[b,c]	370.00	Washington[a]	368.00
Minnesota[c]	402.00	West Virginia[c]	200.00
Mississippi	354.00	Wisconsin	442.72
Missouri	354.00	Wyoming	195.00

[a]California and Washington use their community-property laws in determining what income belongs to the nursing-home spouse and what to the spouse-at-home. Community income is split evenly between the spouses, but only if this benefits the spouse-at-home. After the split, if the spouse-at-home still has less than the indicated standard, the nursing-home spouse is permitted to allocate additional income to bring the income of the spouse-at-home up to the standard. In California, additional amounts of income may be protected to cover alimony or child support ordered by a court.

[b]For residents of Connecticut, Illinois, Michigan, Vermont, and Virginia, the amount that a nursing-home spouse is permitted to protect for his or her spouse-at-home varies by geographic area; the highest amount is shown.

[c]Connecticut, Illinois, Maryland, Michigan, Minnesota, New York, and West Virginia allow additional amounts to be protected if ordered by a court.

[d]In New York, protected amounts may be higher, varying by county, per court order.

[e]Ohio permits protection of $258/month as long as the spouse-at-home's other income is less than $324/month. A spouse-at-home with other income could have as much as $582/month to live on.

SOURCE: National Governors' Association Report.

Personal-Needs Allowance. Not only can a person protect the basic living allowance from the nursing home, but he or she also can keep about $30 a month (depending on the state—see Table 8) for personal needs, such as toiletries, books, and magazines. Don't spend it all in one go!

Unreimbursed Medical Expenses. A nursing-home resident may also keep from the nursing home enough income to pay medical expenses that are not reimbursed by Medicaid or some other third party.

ASSETS LIMITATION TEST

The law in most states used to require people entering a nursing home to pay virtually all their assets to the nursing home before Medicaid would pay anything, even if that meant leaving a spouse-at-home in the poor house. The new Medicare Catastrophic Coverage Act is a little better for some families and much worse for others.

Under the Medicare Catastrophic Coverage Act, a nursing-home resident and his or her spouse-at-home can now protect a minimum of $12,000 or one-half of their combined life savings up to a maximum of $60,000, whichever is more. (States can choose to raise the $12,000 floor, but none have done so at the time of this writing.) Here's how to calculate the amount that can be protected:

1. Total the value of all the nursing-home spouse's assets, his or her spouse-at-home's assets, and jointly held assets. If either spouse has a partial interest in some asset (such as a quarter interest in a rental property), add the value of that interest too.
2. Take one-half the total value of all such combined assets. If the resulting amount is less than $12,000, then $12,000 can be protected. If the amount is more than $60,000, then $60,000 can be protected. If the amount is between $12,000 and $60,000, that amount is what can be protected.

Here are three examples:

Example 5

Your father, who is entering a nursing home, has assets in his name, including CDs and bank accounts, totaling $50,000. Your mother, who is still at home, has assets in her name of $80,000, and they have jointly held assets of $40,000. Total value of all assets is $170,000. One-half would be $85,000. Since that is more than $60,000, your mother could keep the maximum of $60,000, your father would get to keep about $2,000 (the amount listed in Table 10), and the nursing home would get the rest—$108,000—before Medicaid would pay a penny.

Example 6

Your assets at the time you enter a nursing home total $15,000, and the assets of your spouse who is remaining at home come to $5,000, for a $20,000 total. Since one-half is less than the $12,000 minimum, your spouse keeps $12,000, you protect $2,000, and the nursing home gets $6,000.

Example 7

Your nursing-home father has assets of $45,000 and your mother at home has assets of $35,000, for total combined assets of $80,000. One-half is $40,000—so your mother gets $40,000, your father gets $2,000, and the nursing home will get $38,000.

The new assets limitation test applies to married people entering a nursing home on or after September 30, 1989, but does not apply to those already in nursing homes on that date. The new income limitation test applies to all married people in a nursing home or entering one on or after that date.

PROTECTED ASSETS

Even before older people calculate their assets, they can exclude certain assets listed on pages 18–19. In fact, under the Medicare Catastrophic Coverage Act, they can protect their home, household goods and furnishings, personal effects, and a car, *without limitation on their value.* These items are protected *off the top.* For example, if a couple owns a house worth $100,000 and has *other* combined assets of $80,000 (as in Example 7), they could protect the home *and* $42,000 of the remaining assets. As discussed in Chapter 5, wise use of the protections for certain assets can be an important element in planning to avoid the Medicaid trap.

RECORD KEEPING

If a couple must spend some of their assets on nursing-home costs before one of them qualifies for Medicaid, they had better be keeping good records of the value of their assets *at the time one of them is first institutionalized*. Otherwise, they could end up paying more to the nursing home than is legally required.

Let's look back at Example 7. Your nursing-home father would not qualify for Medicaid when he first entered the institution; not until your parents spent $38,000 on the nursing home would he qualify. At the time he applies for Medicaid, after your parents' assets are down to $42,000, Medicaid will want some proof that the assets were $80,000 at the time your father was institutionalized. If your parents can show assets of only $70,000 at that time, they may be required to spend another $5,000 on the nursing home (using one-half of $70,000 instead of one-half of $80,000) before Medicaid will pay anything.

IMPACT OF THE MEDICARE CATASTROPHIC COVERAGE ACT

Is the new law an improvement over prior law? For some, it is. Before, only about $2,000 of a nursing-home spouse's assets (depending on the state) could be protected for the spouse-at-home. Keeping $60,000 is surely better than keeping $2,000.

For others, the new law puts the spouse-at-home in a much more precarious financial position than he or she would have been under the previous law. Before, assets in the name of the spouse not applying for Medicaid generally were protected no matter how much the combined assets totaled. That is no longer the case.

Consider Example 5 again. Under the prior law, in most states your mother would have been entitled to keep the $80,000 of assets in her name, plus at least one-half of the $40,000 jointly held assets (in fact, in many states your mother might have been able to withdraw all $40,000 if it was held in a joint bank account). Instead of getting at least $100,000, as she would have before, your mother is now limited to $60,000.

By making some intelligent transfers of assets between spouses under the old law, your parents might have even been able to keep a much larger share of their combined assets than they can today. Now transfers between spouses are much less helpful (although they should still not be ignored, as discussed in Chapter 5).

In any event, this new law is a panacea for no one. At best, the spouse-at-home can keep only $60,000. For many older Americans, the spouse-at-home will not have enough income to maintain a reasonable standard of living without dipping into the $60,000 in remaining assets. How long will it take to eat up everything worked for during a lifetime? Unfortunately, the answer is still "not long."

The income and asset limitations together can have a devastating impact on many older Americans. To illustrate, let's look at Example 8, which combines Examples 3 and 5.

Example 8

Before your father goes into a nursing home, he and your mother are doing quite well; they've got combined assets of $170,000 and combined monthly income of $2,200—the result of careful planning.

Then your father becomes ill and enters a nursing home. He doesn't qualify for Medicaid until your parents' assets have been spent down to $60,000 (the maximum).

After your father qualifies for Medicaid, your mother would continue to receive her monthly income of $200 and a basic living allowance of $750.20 from your father.

Then your father dies, eliminating his income and the basic living allowance for your mother. Your mother is left with assets of $60,000 and monthly income of $200.

In a situation like Example 8, you can guess what would happen to your mother. The Medicare Catastrophic Coverage Act was aptly named; its effect on your parents may indeed be catastrophic—unless they take steps to protect themselves.

CHAPTER 3 SUMMARY CHECKLIST

As a general rule, older people's income and assets will go to pay nursing-home bills—Medicaid won't pay until their assets are mostly used up.

If a nursing-home resident is *not married*, he or she generally can protect only a limited amount of income and assets and still qualify for Medicaid:

Income

✔ Personal-needs allowance of $30–$70/ month.

✔ Monies spent for health insurance and other medical expenses not covered by Medicaid.

✔ Home-maintenance allowance of about $200/month.

Assets

✔ About $2,000.

✔ Home (regardless of value).

✔ Limited amount of household goods and other personal items up to $2,000 value.

✔ One car up to $4,500 value; no limit on value if used to get to work or medical appointments.

✔ One wedding ring and one engagement ring.

✔ Up to $6,000 equity in property essential for support.

✔ Life insurance with cash surrender value of $1,500.

✔ Burial plot.

✔ Funeral costs up to $1,500/person.

If a nursing-home resident is *married*, the couple generally can protect income and assets as follows:

Income

✔ Basic living allowance for the spouse-at-home up to $1,500/month, based on a complicated formula (beginning September 30, 1989).

✔ Personal-needs allowance for the nursing-home spouse of $30/month.

✔ Unreimbursed medical expenses.

Combined Assets

✔ Half the couple's combined assets up to $60,000.

✔ Home (regardless of value).

✔ Household goods (regardless of value).

✔ Personal effects (regardless of value).

✔ Car (regardless of value).

✔ Up to $6,000 equity in property essential for support.

✔ Life insurance with cash surrender value of $1,500.

✔ Burial plot.

✔ Burial costs up to $1,500/person.

4 | Why Can't Older People Protect Their Nest Egg Just by Giving It Away?

By now the thought may have occurred to you—why shouldn't a nursing-home resident simply get rid of his or her assets right before going into a nursing home? Maybe give them away to his or her kids. Then the nursing-home parent could tell the Medicaid bureaucrats that he or she doesn't have any assets, and Medicaid would pick up the nursing-home tab. If the parent recovered enough to return home, the children would return the assets. If the parent is married, maybe both spouses could give away their assets to their children, who would use those assets to care for the nursing-home parent's spouse-at-home; that arrangement would benefit the parent's spouse-at-home and, eventually, the kids.

Unfortunately, Uncle Sam won't let you or your loved ones protect your assets like this. Transfers of property for less than fair market value made right before a person enters a nursing home are generally not considered valid transfers for Medicaid purposes. In fact, in most cases no transfers are allowed up to *thirty months* in advance of a nursing-home resident's application for Medicaid (or thirty months in advance of the date of entry into a nursing home if the resident has previously applied for and become entitled to Medicaid). Unless you or your loved ones can foresee the future, the transfer-ineligibility rules make planning tough.

For purposes of the transfer-ineligibility rules, transfers include any voluntary transfer of an asset for less than its fair market value. *Involuntary* transfers, such as those resulting from a divorce or foreclosure, do *not* disqualify a Medicaid applicant no matter when the transfers occurred.

Ineligibility Penalty

A transfer of assets within the thirty-month impermissible-transfer period will make a person ineligible for Medicaid for some time.

Example 9

You live in New York and gave your assets to your kids in August 1988. If you apply for Medicaid in July 1991, you should qualify under the assets limitation test; but if you apply in August 1989, the gifts you made the year before would disqualify you from receiving Medicaid assistance.

If a nursing-home resident makes an impermissible transfer within the thirty-month period, he or she will be ineligible for Medicaid for a period (called the ineligibility penalty) determined by:

1. the total uncompensated value of the transferred resources, divided by
2. the average monthly costs for a nursing-home patient in the state or community at the time.

The ineligibility penalty may last no longer than thirty months. Here are two examples of how the penalty works.

Example 10

Six months before your father enters a nursing home, he gives $20,000 to you and his other children. Average nursing-home costs in his state are $2,000/month. Under the new federal law, he would be ineligible for Medicaid for ten months ($20,000 divided by $2,000/month) as a result of the transfer.

Example 11

On January 1, 1989, your father entered a nursing home and transferred his house to your sister. The house was worth $90,000, and the average nursing-home costs in his state were $2,000/month. Taking the $90,000 value and dividing by $2,000/month gives forty-five months. Since the maximum period of ineligibility is thirty months, your father would be ineligible for Medicaid until July 1, 1991 (thirty months later).

There is some question under the Medicare Catastrophic Coverage Act about the date when the ineligibility-penalty period begins. Most likely, the ineligibility penalty will begin to run from the date of the *transfer*. Example 12 shows how this works.

Example 12

On January 1, 1989, your mother transferred $40,000 to her children. She doesn't enter a nursing home and apply for Medicaid until January 1, 1990, twelve months later. Assuming average nursing-home costs of $2,000/month, the ineligibility period would be twenty months ($40,000 divided by $2,000/month), starting January 1, 1989, the date of the *transfer*. By the time your mother entered the nursing home, she would have to wait only eight more months before she could qualify for Medicaid.

However, there is a possibility that states will interpret the law differently, so that the ineligibility penalty will start to run from the date a person enters a nursing home. If that occurs, the story in Example 12 would turn out differently. Once your mother entered a nursing home, she would have to wait the full twenty months, rather than only eight, to qualify for Medicaid.

Regardless of which interpretation wins out, transfers of assets made more than thirty months before your parent applies for Medicaid will not make your parent ineligible for any period.

Example 13

On January 1, 1989, your mother transferred $40,000 to you. On January 1, 1990, she enters a nursing home, but she does not apply for Med-

icaid until August 12, 1991, more than thirty months after the transfer. The previous transfer will not make her ineligible for Medicaid.

Permissible Transfers

Certain transfers, regardless of the date on which they were made, will not make an individual ineligible for Medicaid. A Medicaid applicant will *not* be ineligible if:

- The person transfers a home, whether before or after entering a nursing home, to any of the following:

    1. His or her spouse
    2. Any child who is under twenty-one, blind, or permanently and totally disabled
    3. A sibling who already has some ownership interest in the house and who was residing in the home for at least one year immediately before the person was admitted to a nursing home
    4. Any child who was residing in the house for at least two years immediately before the parent's admission to a nursing home and who provided care for the parent that allowed him or her to stay at home rather than in an institution

- A person transfers any other assets to any of the following:

    1. *After* entering a nursing home, to his or her spouse-at-home
    2. *Before* entering a nursing home, to his or her spouse, but only if the spouse does not transfer the assets to another person (other than back to the parent) for less than full value
    3. To any child who is under twenty-one, blind, or permanently and totally disabled

- A person transfers any *exempt* assets (listed on pages 18–19), other than the house, to anyone.
- A person can prove to the state Medicaid bureaucrats that either:

    1. He or she intended to dispose of the assets for their market value, or
    2. He or she transferred the assets solely for some purpose other than to qualify for Medicaid assistance.

- A person can show that denying him or her Medicaid eligibility would cause an undue hardship.

These exceptions to the transfer-ineligibility rules can be *very* important for you and your loved ones' planning.

Example 14

The day after your father enters a nursing home, and before he applies for Medicaid, he transfers $40,000 to his wife. Because he was already institutionalized, the transfer does not make him ineligible for Medicaid. His wife then transfers the assets to the children, which allows your father to qualify for Medicaid while protecting the assets.

If he made the same transfer one day *before* entering a nursing home, and his wife then transferred the assets, he would be disqualified for Medicaid benefits under the transfer-ineligibility rules.

Example 15

You have been living with and caring for your mother for three years. Without your help, she would have had to go into a nursing home. But you haven't been well lately yourself and can no longer manage for both you and your mother. Reluctantly, you must admit her to a nursing home. If your mother transfers the house into your name, the transfer will protect the house from the nursing home and will not make your mother ineligible for Medicaid.

Example 16

Your mother, who is in a nursing home, transfers her car, some jewelry, and some paintings to you—total value is $15,000. Since all the items were exempt (see pages 18–19), the transfer does not make her ineligible for Medicaid.

The utility of these exceptions to your or your loved ones' planning is discussed in the following chapters.

The transfer rules discussed in this chapter cover transfers of assets made on or after July 1, 1988, *except* for transfers made between spouses. These rules do not apply to transfers between spouses until October 1, 1989. Transfers between spouses prior to that date are governed by existing state rules.

> **NOTE: Under the language of the Medicare Catastrophic Coverage Act, the exception to the transfer-ineligibility rules for assets transferred solely for some purpose other than to qualify for Medicaid assistance conceivably could allow a person to transfer his or her house to any other person at any time. Since possession of a house, which is an exempt asset, does not affect a person's Medicaid eligibility, it could be argued that any transfer would necessarily be for some purpose other than Medicaid qualification. This interpretation of the law would be helpful because you or your loved ones could freely transfer a house, which would then continue to be protected even if it subsequently lost its exempt status.**
>
> **However, reading the law as I've just suggested seems to conflict with the intent of the legislature. For that reason, I have no confidence this argument will be accepted by Medicaid officials or the courts, and I would not recommend relying on this apparent loophole without consulting a lawyer.**

Generally under these rules, no transfers will be allowed up to twenty-four months in advance of an application for Medicaid. States setting different time periods are listed in Table 15.

The thought may cross your mind: Why can't your parent (or you, as an older person) cheat a little by giving away some of his or her assets just before going into a nursing home and forgetting to tell the Medicaid bureaucrats? After all, your parent's assets are minuscule compared with the whole federal Medicaid budget; Uncle Sam will never miss the contribution.

Forget it! While Medicaid generally prohibits only those transfers made within a thirty-month period prior to a Medicaid application, it may go back through an applicant's records (such as tax returns, bank statements, brokerage account statements, etc.) for a much longer period of time, often five years, to check out an application.

For example, your father's federal income tax return for 1984 may show interest income of $5,000. The IRS will conclude that to generate that income, he must have had somewhere in the neighborhood

TABLE 15

Prior to October 1, 1989, Period Within Which Transfers Between Spouses Cannot Be Made to Qualify for Medicaid

STATE	PERIOD WITHIN WHICH TRANSFERS BETWEEN SPOUSES NOT ALLOWED
Alaska	None
California	More than 24 months if state finds evidence that assets were transferred to establish Medicaid eligibility or to reduce nursing-home spouse's share of costs
District of Columbia	None
Idaho	More than 24 months only if state can prove transfer was made to attain Medicaid eligibility
Indiana	5 years
Michigan	1 year
North Carolina	1 year
Oklahoma	5 years if state decides transfer was made to establish Medicaid eligibility
South Dakota	3 years
Washington	None

Note: In almost all states, Medicaid eligibility may not be denied because of transfer of a home to a spouse, no matter when. However, in Louisiana, transfer of the home while the nursing-home spouse is institutionalized makes the home subject to the transfer rules; in Nebraska, transfer of the home is prohibited unless the nursing-home spouse lives there for two years after the transfer. It also should be noted that, in Minnesota, a nursing-home spouse may transfer up to $10,000 to a spouse-at-home at the time of Medicaid application without penalty, so long as the amount transferred does not raise the spouse-at-home's total assets above $10,000.

SOURCE: National Governors' Association Report.

---

of $50,000 of income-generating assets. If those assets don't appear on his Medicaid application, the Medicaid bureaucrats will get suspicious and will start asking a lot of questions. And if Medicaid determines that your father lied on his application, kiss Medicaid funding good-bye. He may also be subject to criminal penalties.

CHAPTER 4 SUMMARY CHECKLIST

In most cases, a person can't give away his or her assets to qualify for Medicaid unless the transfer is made *thirty months* in advance of application for Medicaid. But certain asset transfers do *not* disqualify a person from Medicaid no matter when one applies:

✔ A person can transfer his or her home, before or after entering a nursing home, to any of the following:

1. His or her spouse
2. Any child who is under twenty-one, blind, or permanently and totally disabled
3. A sibling who already has some ownership interest in the house and who was residing in the house for at least one year immediately before the person was admitted to a nursing home
4. Any child who was residing in the house for at least two years immediately before the parent's admission to a nursing home and who provided care for the parent that allowed him or her to stay at home rather than in an institution

✔ A person can transfer any other assets to any of the following:

1. *After* entering a nursing home, to his or her spouse-at-home
2. *Before* entering a nursing home, to his or her spouse, but only if the spouse does not transfer the assets to another person
3. To any child who is under twenty-one, blind, or permanently and totally disabled

✔ A person can transfer any *exempt* assets, other than the house, to anyone.

✔ A person can transfer any assets that he or she intended to dispose of for market value.

✔ A person can transfer any assets solely for a purpose *other than* to qualify for Medicaid.

✔ A person can transfer any assets and still qualify for Medicaid if denying Medicaid would cause him or her an undue hardship.

5 How Can You and Your Family

Avoid the Medicaid Trap?

You may be feeling pretty depressed by this time—and for good reason. Financial tragedy like the one described below can happen to any family.

Gentleman from Maine

> Here I sit, the loneliest man that ever lived. I have admitted my wife of 55 years to a nursing home. She has Alzheimer's and I am caught between a rock and a hard place. I can no longer provide the round-the-clock care she requires, and I will soon be unable to pay the costs of care she now gets, which have exhausted our $160,000 in savings.

Put yourself in that man's place—your life savings disappearing if your spouse needs long-term care.

The politicians have made it as tough as possible to qualify for Medicaid. Prohibited from making most gifts within thirty months of application for Medicaid, a person can't protect his or her assets just by transferring them when he or she is about to enter a nursing home. And without a crystal ball, no one can predict whether an individual will go into a nursing home in thirty months or more.

So is there any practical way to juggle assets to qualify for Medicaid—*before* losing everything? The answer is yes! By following the tips on these pages, an older person or couple can save most or all of their savings, *despite* our lawmakers' best efforts.

Here are the best options:

- Hide money in exempt assets.
- Transfer assets directly to children tax-free.

- Pay children for their help.
- Juggle assets between spouses.
- Pass assets to children through a spouse.
- Transfer a home while retaining a life estate.
- Change wills and title to property.
- Write a durable power of attorney.
- Set up a Medicaid Trust.
- Get a divorce.
- Purchase a long-term-care insurance policy.

By adopting a Medicaid strategy that fits their needs, older persons can avoid the Medicaid trap and keep their savings from the grasp of the nursing home. The options above are discussed in this and subsequent chapters.

Analyze Current Financial Status

Before an older person or couple can choose the best strategy to help protect their savings from a nursing home, they must first make sure they know their present financial status. The following questionnaire is intended to assist in gathering the financial information necessary to design and implement a plan to avoid the catastrophic costs of nursing-home care.

There are seven parts: Assets, Life Insurance, Business Interests, Income, Liabilities, Net Worth, and Gifts.

After an older person or married couple has completed the Medicaid Planning Questionnaire, they will be ready to consider the options available to them to protect their nest egg.

MEDICAID PLANNING QUESTIONNAIRE

Part A: Assets

ASSETS (Give market values where appropriate)	Your Name	Spouse's Name	Joint Names
Residence	$_____	$_____	$_____
Other Real Estate	_____	_____	_____
Cash and Equivalents			
Checking Account(s)	_____	_____	_____
	_____	_____	_____
	_____	_____	_____
Savings Account(s)	_____	_____	_____
	_____	_____	_____
	_____	_____	_____
CDs and Money Market Account(s)	_____	_____	_____
	_____	_____	_____
	_____	_____	_____
Marketable Securities			
Stocks	_____	_____	_____
	_____	_____	_____
	_____	_____	_____
Taxable Bonds	_____	_____	_____
	_____	_____	_____
	_____	_____	_____
Tax-Exempt Bonds	_____	_____	_____
	_____	_____	_____
	_____	_____	_____
Mutual Funds	_____	_____	_____
	_____	_____	_____
	_____	_____	_____
Life-Insurance (from Part B)	_____	_____	_____
Business Interests (from Part C)	_____	_____	_____
Retirement Plans			
Pension/Profit Sharing	_____	_____	_____
IRAs	_____	_____	_____
Personal Property	_____	_____	_____
Other	_____	_____	_____
TOTAL ASSETS	$_____	$_____	$_____
Expectancies (i.e., Inheritances)	_____	_____	_____
TOTAL ASSETS AND EXPECTANCIES	$_____	$_____	$_____

Part B: Life Insurance

Company	Type	Face Value	Cash Value	Insured	Owner	Beneficiary
_____	_____	$_____	$_____	_____	_____	_____
_____	_____	$_____	$_____	_____	_____	_____
_____	_____	$_____	$_____	_____	_____	_____
_____	_____	$_____	$_____	_____	_____	_____
_____	_____	$_____	$_____	_____	_____	_____
_____	_____	$_____	$_____	_____	_____	_____

TOTAL CASH VALUE OF LIFE INSURANCE

You $_____   Your Spouse $_____

(Include these amounts on Life Insurance line in Part A)

Part C: Business Interests

Name of Business _____

Percentage of Interest Owned by
You _____%   Your Spouse _____%   Jointly _____%

Percentage Owned by Children
Name _____   _____%
Name _____   _____%
Name _____   _____%

Tax Basis of Business (if you know) $_____

Book Value of Business (if you know) $_____

YOUR ESTIMATE OF PRESENT VALUE OF BUSINESS
You $_____   Your Spouse $_____   Jointly $_____

(Include these amounts on Business Interests line in Part A)

Part D: Income

	Your Monthly Income	Spouse's Monthly Income	Total Monthly Income
Net Salary or Wages ("Take-Home Pay")	$_____	$_____	$_____
Social Security Benefits	_____	_____	_____
Retirement Benefits	_____	_____	_____
Interest	_____	_____	_____
Dividends	_____	_____	_____
Other	_____	_____	_____
TOTAL INCOME	$_____	$_____	$_____

Part E: Liabilities

LIABILITIES (Give outstanding balances)	Your Name	Spouse's Name	Joint Names
Residence			
Primary Mortgage	$	$	$
Second Mortgage			
Other Real Estate Mortgages			
Personal Loans			
Income Taxes			
Other Debts			
TOTAL LIABILITIES	$	$	$

Part F: Net Worth

	Your Name	Spouse's Name	Joint Names
Total Assets (from Part A) minus	$	$	$
Total Liabilities (from Part E)			
NET WORTH (Assets minus liabilities)	$	$	$

Part G: Gifts

(Gifts made in excess of $10,000/year to an individual other than your spouse)

Recipient _____ Date _____ Amount $ _____
Recipient _____ Date _____ Amount $ _____
Recipient _____ Date _____ Amount $ _____
Recipient _____ Date _____ Amount $ _____

Hide Money in Exempt Assets

As discussed in Chapter 3, certain assets are removed from Medicaid's reach. By putting money into these exempt assets, an elderly person or couple can preserve their savings.

HOUSE

The most significant exemption is for a personal residence. Right now, all but one state, Missouri, allow a nursing-home resident to exclude the entire value of his or her house, and even in Missouri the whole value of the house will be protected after October 1, 1989; many states permit the exclusion to last for a virtually unlimited period. As a result of this exemption, an elderly person's or couple's house can be a treasure chest for their savings.

If they already own a home but it has a mortgage, they can take money from their savings account, cash in a CD, or sell some stock to pay off the loan. This is not considered a prohibited transfer of assets, so they can do this at any time. By paying off a mortgage, they can magically change assets like cash, which would be lost to a nursing home, into assets that can't be touched. Since they can exclude the entire value of their house whether it's got a large mortgage or no mortgage, they may as well pay off the mortgage.

They can also hide money in their house by making improvements, such as adding a family room, putting on a new roof, or redoing their kitchen. Again, by pouring money into their home, they can protect assets from the nursing home's grasp and improve their life-style as well.

If they don't own a home, they could think about buying one. The same principle applies—take assets that could be reached by the nursing home and make them unreachable by "sheltering" them in a house. And again, a person or couple can wait until nursing-home admission is imminent, because buying a home is not a transfer that is penalized under the transfer-ineligibility rules. That way, if a person or couple really doesn't want a home, they won't have to buy one until they're sure they will benefit by qualifying for Medicaid.

Since there's no limit on the value of a house that they can buy, they may be able to hide most or all of their assets with this one simple technique. This is a giant loophole, which they should feel free to take advantage of. Whether the house they buy costs $50,000 or $200,000 makes no difference; in all but one state, it is protected from the reach of the nursing home.

If they later need the cash for some emergency, they can always get to it by taking out a mortgage, a home equity loan, or some other loan against the equity in the house. Although it's not as liquid an asset as cash, it isn't totally inaccessible.

Hiding money in a house works best if an older person has a spouse or dependent relative at home. If the person is unmarried and has no dependents at home, the house may lose its immunity from the nursing home's reach. As shown in Table 11, a number of states limit the home exclusion for unmarried nursing-home residents to a period from six months to a year; in many states, a home may lose its protection as soon as it becomes clear to a physician that the nursing-home resident will never recover enough to return.

Even if there is a spouse or dependent relative at home, further precautions will have to be taken in order to save the house—and all the money hidden in it. While the house will remain exempt from the nursing home's grasp as long as a spouse (or dependent relative) continues to live in it, regardless of whose name is on the title, consider what happens if the spouse (or dependent relative) dies or moves out. If the house is in the nursing-home resident's name, or held jointly with a spouse (see the discussion of how to deal with jointly held property in the next chapter), the house will belong solely to the nursing-home resident when his or her spouse dies, and since no spouse (or dependent relative) would be living there, it could then lose its protection. In that event, the nursing-home resident's Medicaid coverage would cease (or just not begin); the house would be sold; and the proceeds would be used to pay the resident's bills.

To avoid this situation, nursing-home residents should transfer the house to their spouse-at-home as soon as they go into a nursing home (or before, if entry becomes apparent), and the spouse should have a will leaving the house to the couple's children or other chosen heirs. The heirs will receive the house under the spouse's will, rather than have it end up sold to pay nursing-home bills.

Such transfers can't be planned too far in advance, and an important tool in such planning is a "durable power of attorney" (the subject of Chapter 7). Say both your parents are still alive and married. You can't predict which one might have to enter a nursing home first. Unfortunately, once a person becommes incompetent (so often the reason that nursing-home care is needed), that person can no longer legally transfer real estate. If your home-owning parent fails to transfer the home before he or she becomes incompetent (or if the house remains jointly owned), the chance to protect the house from nursing-home costs will have been lost—*unless* the parent has a durable power of attorney.

One last note to keep in mind: Whereas it may be advisable for an older couple to pay off a mortgage or make improvements to a home, buying a house as a repository for assets can be more problematic, particularly if the couple waits until one of them is about to enter a nursing home. Someone caring for a loved one with Alzheimer's, for example, is likely to be emotionally and physically exhausted and will probably not have the energy or will to cope with buying a house as well. Buying a home creates its own stress, requiring dealings with financial institutions, real estate agents, and attorneys.

HOUSEHOLD GOODS AND PERSONAL ITEMS

All states allow a nursing-home resident to protect some household goods and personal items, such as furniture and clothing. If the person is married, household goods, a car, and personal effects are protected *without regard to their value!*

This exemption offers an excellent way to "hide" assets. Is it time to buy a new refrigerator? Is the stove on its last legs? Instead of "making do," this may be the time to buy replacements.

The exemption for household goods and personal items may be used creatively to protect many assets. For example, oriental rugs or paintings that appreciate in value may be worthwhile investments that add beauty and hide assets at the same time.

WEDDING AND ENGAGEMENT RINGS

Generally, states allow a person to protect one wedding ring and one engagement ring. Under the new Medicare Catastrophic Coverage Act, if a nursing-home resident is married, he or she can probably protect any number of rings or other pieces of jewelry. Here's another loophole that a nursing-home resident may want to consider. He or she could buy a brand-new—and expensive—ring right before going into a nursing home. After all, the law doesn't limit this exclusion to rings purchased at the time of a wedding or engagement. Cashing in assets that can be claimed by the nursing home, in order to buy a ring, does not fall under rules prohibiting transfer of assets. So one can take advantage of this loophole at any time.

On the downside, rings may depreciate over time, leaving the spouse-at-home or heirs without the full value of the nursing-home resident's assets. For this reason, hiding money in rings may not be the best alternative.

PROPERTY ESSENTIAL TO SUPPORT

As discussed on pages 18–19 and presented in Table 12, almost all states allow an unmarried nursing-home resident to protect real estate and personal property that is essential to his or her support up to an equity value of $6,000 if the property produces a net annual income of at least 6 percent of the excluded equity. The same protection is available to married couples in every state. Income-producing property, such as rental units or farmland, may be covered. Some planners have even argued that stocks and bonds may be covered in certain situations if the person is living off the income, although the Medicaid bureaucrats and courts have not yet said so.

The same principle applies here as it did above. If the person has a small productive family business, he or she should consider protecting assets by upgrading equipment and making other necessary improvements.

FAMILY BURIAL PLOTS

After spending their life savings on long-term nursing-home care, some older Americans have been left without enough even for a proper burial. The nursing-home resident can avoid this sad conclusion by prepaying for burial plots (no dollar limit) and funeral costs (up to $1,500/person).

But he or she shouldn't go overboard "burying" money in cemetery plots because, unlike a house, oriental rugs, or other household goods, a burial plot cannot be passed on to a spouse or heirs.

Example 17

> At the time your father enters a nursing home, he and your mother have combined assets of $200,000, excluding the value of their house. He immediately transfers the home into your mother's name. The house has an $80,000 mortgage, which they pay off. Your mother buys a new car for cash, paying $10,000. She also buys a few things for the house, including an oriental rug, for a $15,000 total cost. Finally, she buys burial plots and prepays burial costs for your father and herself, for a total of $5,000.
>
> These expenses reduce your parents' combined nonexempt assets to $90,000. Your mother can keep one-half of that amount, or $45,000; your father gets to keep $2,000; and the nursing home will get $43,000 before Medicaid will begin to pay your father's bills. By taking these steps, your parents were able *legally* to protect $100,000, which otherwise would have disappeared.

Although it may go against your grain to take such advantage of loopholes in the law, remember that "hiding" assets in these exclusions may be the best way for a nursing-home resident to protect at least a portion of the family nest egg for his or her spouse and children.

Transfer Assets Directly to Children, Other Relatives, or Friends

It is possible to transfer *exempt* assets other than a house (see the list on pages 18–19) to *anyone* at *any time* without penalty under the transfer-ineligibility rules. As shown in Example 16, by transferring exempt assets to children, other relatives, or friends (but not between spouses), older persons can get those assets out of their names—and out of the nursing home's grasp.

And as discussed later in this chapter, Uncle Sam gives older persons a tax break that helps them use this transfer technique to protect assets. Most people can transfer all their assets without paying any additional tax.

Why worry about transferring exempt assets? After all, since they're exempt they won't be included as assets for Medicaid purposes. But they may not always be exempt, as Example 18 demonstrates.

Example 18

Your mother is in a nursing home. She has paintings and jewelry worth $15,000. While your father is alive, all of that is exempt. But should he die, only $2,000 would remain exempt (see page 18 and Table 12) and the rest would have to be sold to pay your mother's nursing-home costs.

Had your mother transferred her assets to you while they were exempt, with her husband alive, they would have been protected even after he passed away. Then, if she recovered enough to return home, you could return the assets.

Other assets that are not exempt under the Medicaid rules may also be transferred. Transfers made thirty months or more before a person enters a nursing home will not be counted by Medicaid. But that thirty-month period makes transfers of nonexempt assets unappealing to most people as a technique to protect assets. How many people are comfortable giving away their money and property long before they know if they will even need long-term care?

Some people give all their assets to their children with the expectation or unwritten understanding that the children will take care of them. While that can be an effective way to keep assets from the nursing home, it could put the parents' financial security in jeopardy. All too often, parents have given assets to children who later turn their backs on them. Even if the children are well-meaning, they may have spent the money for some purpose, perhaps to pay off their own emergency medical bills, and when the parents need help it's just not available. If parents don't want to make themselves dependent on their kids or to put themselves at risk, they should not give away assets they need to live on.

Parents' gifts to their children just to beat Medicaid, with the understanding that the assets are really to be used for the parents' benefit, could be considered a life-care contract, which would constitute an asset of the parents with a value that could disqualify them from receiving Medicaid. And in rare circumstances, the transfer of assets to children with such an "understanding" could be considered Medicaid and/or tax fraud, exposing the parents to possible criminal penalties.

For all these reasons, parents should be careful when considering whether to use gifts to children or others as a technique to keep their savings from the nursing home.

Pay Children for Their Help

Let's say that you have been helping your widowed mother with a variety of chores—driving her to the store, doing her banking, preparing meals. Maybe you have even moved into her house to provide full-time care. Your parent could transfer assets without worrying about the transfer prohibition rules by paying you for services rendered.

This can be a very helpful technique if used carefully—Medicaid personnel are likely to scrutinize payments to children. Only reasonable payments can be made. A parent can't pay a child $2,000 each time the child drives him or her to the store and expect Medicaid to overlook it. But if full-time care provided at home costs $40,000 per year in your area, a child providing the same services could be fairly compensated that same amount.

Of course, most children helping their parents do so without any expectation of payment. And that's as it should be. But if a parent is about to go into a nursing home, consider using a portion of assets to pay a reasonable amount for services that have been rendered.

Juggle Assets Between Spouses

This remains an important planning tool, although Congress has taken steps to undercut its utility.

Before the new Medicare Catastrophic Coverage Act, "equalizing assets" between spouses was the first planning technique recommended for married couples. It would ensure that they could preserve *at least one-half of their combined life savings.* By putting one-half of a couple's assets in the name of one spouse and one-half in the other spouse's name, at least one spouse's half of the total assets would be protected if the other went into a nursing home.

Now, equalizing assets is much less helpful. Under the new law, a couple's assets are all lumped together and then divided, so transferring assets from one spouse to another spouse, in and of itself, won't protect their assets while both are living.

Does this mean that there is no longer any reason to juggle assets between spouses? The answer is no! And the reason is simple: If a nursing-home spouse keeps assets in his or her name, and the spouse-at-home dies first, the nursing-home spouse will end up unnecessarily losing all but $2,000 of his or her assets, *including* the $60,000 that the law allowed the spouse-at-home to retain while he or she was living.

Example 19

At the time your father enters a nursing home, he and your mother have total assets of $170,000—$150,000 in your father's name and $20,000 in the name of your mother. Your father and mother are able to protect a total of $62,000 under the assets limitation test for married individuals (see page 27).

Two years after your father enters the nursing home, he has $100,000 left in his name ($50,000 was spent on nursing-home costs), and your mother has $15,000 left in her name. Then your mother dies. Since your father is no longer married, the assets limitation test for unmarried individuals, rather than that for married individuals, takes over. Now your father is allowed to keep only about $2,000 of assets in his name, and your mother's heirs will receive under her will the $15,000 that was in her name at the time of her death. In other words, $17,000 is the total of your parents' life savings that would be protected from a nursing home; over $150,000 would be lost. If your father recovered enough to return home, he would return to a life of poverty.

This example shows a common mistake that can cost a family thousands of dollars. Look at Example 20 to see what should have been done.

Example 20

At the time your father enters a nursing home, he and your mother have total assets of $170,000; your father doesn't qualify for Medicaid. As soon as he enters, he transfers everything into your mother's name. That transfer won't help him qualify for Medicaid immediately, but it will help later, with the same events as in Example 19.

Two years after he enters the nursing home, your mother has $120,000 left in her name; the rest went toward payment of nursing-home bills. Then she dies. All $120,000 would transfer to her children (or other named beneficiaries) under your mother's will (assuming she changed it; see Chapter 6); your father would then qualify for Medicaid, which would pick up the remaining nursing-home costs. If your father subsequently recovered enough to return home, the children could return his assets.

You can see immediately why a nursing-home parent should shift assets to his or her spouse-at-home under the new law. Failing to do that can be a very costly mistake.

Don't worry about any tax implications. As will be discussed shortly, transfers to a spouse, no matter how much, can be made tax-free.

A couple can (and in most cases should) wait to juggle assets between themselves until one of them enters a nursing home, because no transfer-limitation period applies to any assets transferred between spouses after one spouse enters a nursing home.

Pass Assets to Children Through a Spouse

If parents trust their children to take care of them, they should be able to protect any of their assets by passing them through a spouse to children. Here is an example of how this technique works:

Example 21

Your parents have combined assets of $200,000. Right after your father enters a nursing home, he transfers everything to your mother. Then, before your father applies for Medicaid, your mother transfers $150,000 to her three children.

In this situation, your mother will be able to protect $25,000 of the remaining funds (one-half of the $50,000 she retained), your father keeps $2,000, and the nursing home gets $23,000. The $150,000 transferred to the kids cannot be touched.

In this way, parents are able to transfer assets to children without running afoul of the transfer-ineligibility rules. The transfer of assets from a nursing-home spouse to a spouse-at-home after the nursing-home spouse enters a nursing home is a permissible transfer that does not cause the nursing-home spouse to become ineligible; and the spouse-at-home, who is not applying for Medicaid, can then transfer the assets to anyone else without penalty.

Example 22 shows what the result would be if a nursing-home parent tried to transfer even some of his or her assets directly to a child, without passing them through a spouse.

Example 22

Your mother transfers her nonexempt assets of $100,000 to you immediately after entering a nursing home. She will be ineligible for Medicaid for the maximum thirty-month period. Assuming average nursing-home costs of $2,000/month, you will have paid all but $40,000 of her $100,000 transfer in nursing-home costs before she is eligible for Medicaid.

The timing of transfers to children through a spouse is crucial. These transfers must be made *after* the nursing-home spouse enters a nursing home but *before* the nursing-home spouse applies for Medicaid. If a parent transfers assets to a spouse *before* going into a nursing home, and the spouse tries to pass the assets to a child, the parent's transfer *will* be subject to the thirty-month impermissible-transfer period.

Example 23

Your father has assets of $60,000 in his name, and your mother has no assets in her name. Two weeks *before* your father enters a nursing home, he transfers everything into your mother's name. That transfer, by itself, would not affect his Medicaid eligibility. Your mother would protect $30,000 (one-half of their total combined assets), your father would protect $2,000, and the nursing home would receive $28,000.

But if your mother transfers the $60,000 to the children, your father's original transfer to your mother would suddenly run afoul of the transfer-ineligibility rules. Assuming average nursing-home costs of $2,000/month, he would not qualify for Medicaid for the thirty-month maximum ineligibility penalty period, forcing your parents to lose the entire $60,000.

Had your father waited a couple of weeks to transfer his assets, until just *after* he entered a nursing home, neither that transfer nor the subsequent transfer by your mother to the children would have made him ineligible for Medicaid (as long as the transfers were made before he applied for Medicaid). In that case, all $60,000 would have been protected.

The chief benefit of passing assets through a spouse to children, rather than directly to children, is that the thirty-month impermissible-transfer period won't apply. That means parents can wait until one of them actually must enter a nursing home before taking action. Because they don't have to make transfers far in advance, they minimize the risk of putting themselves at the mercy of their children.

Still, parents should consider this technique only if they have a great deal of faith that their children *will* help them financially if need be. If they do, this planning technique can be, literally, a lifesaver for the spouse-at-home.

Transfer a Home While Retaining a Life Estate

Here's another option for a parent who wants to protect at least a portion of the equity in a house, but also wants to be sure that he or she will be able to live there as long as possible.

Example 24

Your father is widowed, and his primary asset is his house. He is healthy now, but he is concerned about losing his house due to long-term-care costs in the future. He doesn't want to place himself in jeopardy by transferring the house outright to his children at this point in his life. What can he do?

Your father could transfer a so-called remainder interest in the home to his children, keeping a "life estate" for himself. That means he would retain a legal right to live in the house during his lifetime, but his children would own the home after he dies.

If your father enters a nursing home before he dies, the value of the "life estate" probably would be counted in his assets, but that amount would be less than the market value of the entire ownership of the house.

This technique will not protect the entire value of a parent's home. A life estate has a value, which may be calculated using the American Experience Tables of Mortality (available at your local library). The value of the life estate will be less than the market value of the home. For example, if the market value of the house is $100,000, a life estate may be worth $50,000, depending on the parent's age. If the parent goes into a nursing home, that lesser amount, not the entire $100,000 market value, would be counted in his or her assets.

Retaining a life estate while transferring a remainder interest can be a valuable planning tool for a parent, particularly if he or she is unmarried and does not want to relinquish his or her right to live in the house. But this technique can be complicated and requires the help of an experienced attorney.

Be Aware of the Tax Laws

In almost all cases discussed in this book, shifting assets won't affect the amount of taxes parents or their children will pay. Questions come up most often about three types of federal taxes: (1) gift or transfer taxes; (2) capital gains taxes; and (3) income taxes.

GIFT OR TRANSFER TAXES

Gift taxes (also called transfer taxes) are paid only by the donor of a gift, not the recipient (probably the donor's spouse or children in this case). And unless the donor is planning to give away $600,000 or more during his or her lifetime, no federal gift or transfer taxes will ever have to be paid by anyone.

The federal law provides a unified transfer-tax exemption which allows any person to make $600,000 worth of gifts during his or her lifetime without paying any transfer or gift tax. In addition, a person can make unlimited gifts to his or her spouse free of gift or transfer tax (under the unlimited marital deduction). And anyone can make gifts of up to $10,000/person each year free of federal gift

or transfer taxes without using up even a penny of his or her $600,000 lifetime gift-tax exemption.

Example 25

Your father and mother are both living and have four children. If they each give $10,000 gifts to each child, they could get rid of as much as $80,000 each year tax-free without using any of the $600,000 lifetime gift-tax exemption available to each of them.

Look back at Example 21. Your father's transfer to your mother, since it is a gift from one spouse to another, would be completely free of any transfer or gift tax. Your mother's transfer of $150,000 to her three children would also be free of gift or transfer tax: three $10,000 gifts (to each child) would come under the annual gift-tax exclusion, and $120,000 could come under your mother's $600,000 unified transfer-tax exemption.

As you can see, chances are that gift or transfer taxes will have absolutely no effect on a person's planning to avoid the catastrophic costs of long-term care.

CAPITAL GAINS TAXES

In rare situations, federal capital gains taxes may impact on a person's planning. Generally, capital gains taxes are paid on the appreciated value of an item when it is sold. Here is an example of how these taxes work:

Example 26

Your mother bought shares of stock for $2,000 (called the basis) in 1950 and has held them ever since; today they're worth $50,000. If she sells the shares, she'll pay capital gains tax on $48,000 (the increased value).

Example 27 shows how the capital gains taxes are reduced or even completely avoided if your mother, in the above example, holds the shares until she dies.

Example 27

Your mother bought shares of stock in 1950 for $2,000 and today those shares are worth $50,000. Your mother died recently, leaving the stock to her children, who sell it for $50,000. The children will pay no capital gains tax because, when the shares of stock passed to the children on your mother's death, the "basis" of the shares was increased from $2,000 to $50,000.

The basis does *not* increase if a person transfers appreciated stock (or other items) during his or her lifetime. Taking Example 27, had your mother transferred the stock to her children during her lifetime, her children would get her $2,000 basis, not a "step-up" to a $50,000 basis. If her children were to sell the stock ten years later for $60,000, they would pay capital gains tax on $58,000 ($60,000 minus $2,000) rather than on $10,000 ($60,000 minus $50,000).

Before people start shifting assets, they should consider possible implications of the capital gains tax. In situations where older Americans have significantly appreciated assets, they and their families may be much better off financially just holding on to them.

INCOME TAXES

If parents transfer assets to their children, the children will not pay any income tax on receiving the assets. The only income tax they eventually will pay is on any income produced from the transferred assets.

Example 28

Your parents transfer $100,000 in cash to you. You will pay no income tax when you receive the money. You then invest the cash in CDs yielding 8 percent—$8,000 in annual interest. That interest is added to your income and will be taxed.

As long as people are aware of the tax rules, they should be able to develop a strategy to protect their savings without paying any additional taxes.

Don't Fall for Special Nursing-Home Requirements

Some nursing homes try to require the children of nursing-home patients to pay their parent's bills even though the parent could qualify for Medicaid. The nursing home would charge the family *more* than Medicaid would pay for the parent's care. If the children refuse, they are told that their parent cannot enter or remain in the nursing home. What

good is planning to protect assets if the nursing home can require children to pay for their parent's bills and completely avoid the Medicaid rules?

The Medicaid laws do *not* require children to pay their parent's nursing-home bills. So can a nursing home legally condition a parent's admission or continued stay on the children's agreement to pay all or a part of their parent's bills? The answer is probably no if the nursing home participates in the Medicaid program.

Federal law makes it a crime for the nursing home to ask the children for, or to receive from them, any payment when:

- The payment is required as a precondition to their parent's admission.
- The payment is required for their parent's continued stay in the nursing home.

There have not been many lawsuits over nursing homes requiring children to pay parents' bills. Generally, the children, unaware that they don't have to dissipate their own assets, go ahead and make the payments—even if it creates significant hardship for the family. But in one recent New York case, the family of a nursing-home patient took the nursing home to court and won.

In that case, Robert Snook signed an agreement with a nursing home that committed him to pay $95.00/day for his mother's care for eighteen months. The nursing home, which participated in the Medicaid program, otherwise would have received much less from Medicaid. After several months, Robert felt that he could no longer make the payments and applied for Medicaid on his mother's behalf. The nursing home objected and went to court to force him to make the payments under the terms of his contract.

The court ruled that the contract was illegal and could not be enforced. Noting that a federal regulation requires nursing homes participating in the Medicaid program to "accept, as payment in full, the amounts paid by [Medicaid]," the court explained that this regulation was "designed as a protection against the misfortune" of older Americans and their families. According to the court, the Medicaid payment to the nursing home should represent "the reasonable cost or reasonable charges" for the services provided, and nursing homes should not be permitted to condition admission or continued stay upon higher payments by family members.

If you already have a parent in a nursing home

that accepts Medicaid and have signed an agreement like the one Robert Snook signed, you may have the right to stop making payments—without any harm coming to your parent. And, if you haven't yet agreed to supplement your parent's Medicaid payments, don't—at least not until you've consulted with an attorney who can advise you about your rights.

Apply for Medicaid

After a person has taken steps to protect his or her assets, and following the expiration of any transfer-ineligibility period, the person will be ready to apply for Medicaid.

The first step to apply for Medicaid is to complete a form that, in most states, can be procured from a local welfare or public health or Social Security office. Many hospitals have a social worker on staff who can help direct one to the right place for an application and who will even give advice on filling it out.

The forms differ in each state. Often they look complicated and involved. Don't be scared off by the application! Fill out as much as you can and submit it as quickly as possible. The sooner a parent or child gets the application in, the sooner the patient may begin to collect.

The forms generally seek information concerning a nursing-home patient's age, income, assets, citizenship, residency, personal circumstances (such as employment and family members), disability if any, and medical expenses.

After the person has submitted the form, someone from Medicaid will interview the person, his or her spouse, and/or any children. Proof of the information requested in the application should be brought to the interview. For example, to show income, pay stubs, W-2s, or similar information will be required; to show assets, copies of items like bank and money market statements may be necessary. All information provided in the application and the interview is strictly confidential.

After reviewing the application and considering the interview, Medicaid will decide whether the applicant needs nursing-home care and is eligible for Medicaid. The state sets a time limit—usually forty-five to sixty days—within which Medicaid must make a decision. Of course, the quicker Medicaid receives the necessary information, the faster the applicant should get a response.

If the applicant is *approved*, his or her Medicaid funding should begin promptly. In fact, if he or she entered a nursing home while waiting for Medicaid's decision and paid out of his or her own pocket for a period of time, the patient should be able to get a refund from the nursing home of part or all of those prior payments.

If Medicaid *denies* a person's application, that person has a right to appeal. Depending on the rules in the state, he or she may appeal to a state hearing officer, a state medical board, and/or a state court. In the case of an appeal, Medicaid must provide a form and will help the applicant fill it out. But if a person has been denied, he or she should probably get legal help with the appeal. Don't delay. Ask Medicaid how much time you or your loved one has to appeal. If you miss the deadline (which varies from state to state, usually from ten to ninety days), you (or your loved one) may lose your right to appeal.

CHAPTER 5 SUMMARY CHECKLIST

Options for Preserving Assets

Place Money in Exempt Assets

- ✔ Pay off home mortgage.

- ✔ Make necessary home improvements.

- ✔ Buy needed household goods and/or personal effects.

- ✔ Buy household goods and/or personal effects that will appreciate.

- ✔ Upgrade equipment for a small productive family business.

- ✔ Set aside funds for burial plots and funeral costs.

Transfer Assets to Children, Spouse, and/or Others

- ✔ Make gifts of exempt assets to children or others whom you trust to help you in a financial emergency.

- ✔ Make gifts of nonexempt assets directly to children or others more than thirty months before entering a nursing home.

✔ Transfer house into the name of your spouse-at-home before or after entering a nursing home.

✔ Shift other assets to your spouse-at-home *after* you have entered a nursing home.

✔ Pass assets to your children through a spouse-at-home *after* you have entered a nursing home.

✔ Pay children for services they have provided.

✔ Optionally, transfer house to children while retaining a life estate.

Be Aware of Tax Laws

Avoid Special Nursing-Home Requirements

✔ Children of a nursing-home parent cannot be required to pay the bills as a precondition of a parent's admission into a nursing home that accepts Medicaid patients.

✔ Children of a nursing-home parent cannot be required to pay the bills as a condition of a parent's continued stay in a nursing home that accepts Medicaid patients.

6 | Changing One's Will and

Title to Property

The techniques discussed so far can shield money and property from the grasp of a nursing home. We have learned that older persons can protect assets by changing them into exempt assets or transferring them between themselves and to others. But all that planning may be for naught if a person fails to change his or her will and title to property.

Wills

Look back at Example 20. In that example, your father transferred all his assets into your mother's name after he entered a nursing home. Then your mother died, leaving the assets to her children, thereby protecting those assets from the nursing home. But if your mother's will had left everything to *your father*, and if she had failed to change it after your father entered a nursing home, the end of this story would change completely!

Example 29

When your father entered a nursing home, he transferred his cash and house to your mother, in order to protect them from the nursing home. Two years after he entered the nursing home, your mother dies.

Many years earlier, your father and mother each made wills leaving everything to each other. After your father went into a nursing home, your mother forgot to change her will. When she dies, the assets don't go to her children, as your parents had planned. All her assets go to your father

under your mother's will—and then to the nursing home.

All the planning in the world is worthless if people forget to change their wills. As soon as someone named as a beneficiary enters a nursing home, that person should be removed from the will. Otherwise, the bequest will end up going to the nursing home.

Title to Property

How is your or your loved one's home titled? What about checking and savings accounts, stocks, CDs, and money markets? For most married couples, many, if not all, of their assets are jointly held. People may even hold assets jointly with their child or friend. Although there are a lot of benefits to owning property jointly, it can turn out to be the *worst* option when Medicaid looms.

WHAT IS JOINT OWNERSHIP?

Any person together with someone else, usually a spouse or child, may own property jointly with a right of survivorship. This means that, while both owners are alive, both own and control the property. When one owner dies, that person's interest in the property is automatically transferred to the surviving co-owner.

For example, if your mother and father have a joint and survivorship bank account, when your father dies the entire account will belong to your mother. Of course, if your mother dies first, the account is your father's.

All sorts of property can be held jointly with a right of survivorship. Homes, bank accounts, CDs, and stocks typically are owned jointly with a right of survivorship.

WHY IS JOINT OWNERSHIP SO POPULAR?

The main reason so many people like joint ownership with a right of survivorship is that it avoids probate. A generation in this country grew up on the notion that they should avoid probate at all costs, and owning assets jointly with a right of survivorship simply and inexpensively accomplishes that goal.

On the death of one spouse, the assets are shifted automatically to the other. Because transfers under a right of survivorship take precedence over a will, they do not go through probate.

Of course, there are other reasons people own assets jointly. Not the least is a feeling that spouses are equal and should be treated that way.

WHAT'S WRONG WITH JOINT OWNERSHIP WHEN IT COMES TO MEDICAID?

Owning property jointly can cause older persons to lose *everything* to a nursing home.

Example 30

At the time your mother enters a nursing home, she and your father have total assets (including a home) of $200,000. All of the money is held jointly with a right of survivorship.

Shortly after your mother enters the nursing home, and before your parents have a chance to start juggling their assets, your father dies. All the jointly held assets transfer automatically to your mother. Your mother won't qualify for Medicaid until virtually all of those assets are gone.

Because joint and survivorship ownership of property takes precedence over a will, all jointly held assets would pass to your mother even if your father's will left everything to the children. As this example shows, it's not sufficient just to change a will.

Of course, your parents could have taken the advice given in Chapter 5 and transferred everything out of joint and survivorship ownership into your father's name alone once your mother entered a nursing home; that would have avoided a total financial loss. In fact, your father probably could have emptied their joint bank accounts without worrying about the transfer-ineligibility rules. But people don't always have time to do that. Your father may die before he gets around to make the transfers—after all, if your mother goes into a nursing home, transferring assets probably won't be at the top of your parents' list of priorities. And if your mother becomes incapacitated, transferring assets could be delayed or prevented entirely.

Had your parents each owned one-half of the assets, they would at least have saved some of their estate. Using Example 30, if $100,000 had been in your mother's name and $100,000 in your father's name, your father's half could have passed to the children under his will, leaving only your mother's half to finance nursing-home costs.

In fact, joint and survivorship ownership can be disastrous when it comes to Medicaid planning, because joint owners run the risk of losing everything if *either one* goes into a nursing home. In the above example, if all your parents' assets were in your mother's name, there would be a fifty-fifty chance that your father, not your mother, would be the one to need long-term nursing care; the same odds would apply if all the assets were in your father's name. With joint and survivorship ownership, your parents can lose everything *regardless* of who enters a nursing home first.

There are two other potentially serious problems with joint and survivorship ownership that people should think about before deciding how to handle their assets.

Right to Control the Asset. Each person named on a joint and survivorship asset owns it. For example, if your father puts your or a friend's name on his house deed or bank account, that property is 50 percent yours or the friend's. Your father's co-owner has a right to live in the house or to take money from the account. Your father can't sell a house jointly titled with someone else without the co-owner's approval and signature. All this can create problems if the co-owner is not available or refuses to cooperate.

Precedence over a Will. Let's say your mother's estate consists of a $100,000 bank account. She has three children, and her will says everything she owns should be divided equally among the children after she dies. One child offers to help your mother pay bills and handle her banking, so she puts that child's name on the bank account. When your mother dies, that one child may get *everything* in the account, rather than one-third as your mother had intended; the other kids may be left with nothing.

People should not ignore the way they hold property. Many older people don't even know how their assets are titled. Yet this can have a tremendous impact on their financial stability should one of them require long-term nursing care. They should consider their priorities and select the type of ownership that is best for them.

CHAPTER 6 SUMMARY CHECKLIST

The benefits from planning may be lost by failing to change wills or title to property. You or your loved ones should:

- ✔ Not leave assets in a will to someone who is already in a nursing home.

- ✔ Consider equalizing at least a portion of the assets.

- ✔ Consider alternatives to owning a home, bank accounts, and other assets jointly with rights of survivorship.

- ✔ Transfer all jointly held assets into the name of the spouse-at-home once the other spouse has entered a nursing home.

7 A Durable Power of Attorney: The Most Important Planning Tool

Making a durable power of attorney is the single most important thing most people can do to avoid the Medicaid trap and protect their savings. Yet most people have never even heard of it.

A durable power of attorney can *guarantee* that you and your loved ones will not spend any more than about $60,000 (two and one-half years' costs) on a nursing home. *No one should ever lose more!*

Example 31

Your father is incapacitated in an auto accident and must be admitted to a nursing home. At the time of his accident, he has assets worth $150,000.

As soon as he enters the nursing home, he transfers all but $60,000 of his assets—enough to pay the nursing-home costs for two and one-half years—to you.

Two and one-half years later, when the assets transfer-ineligibility period is met, he can qualify for Medicaid. He was able to protect $90,000 of his assets.

This example, drawing upon techniques already discussed, demonstrates how people can preserve their nest egg, even if they haven't started shifting assets before one enters a nursing home. By transferring assets upon entering an institution and then waiting for the ineligibility period—two and one-half years—to expire, a person should be able to avoid losing any more than the costs incurred in that period.

This sounds great, except that many people aren't *able* to transfer property when they enter a nursing home. Maybe they're so physically or mentally impaired that they can't legally make a valid transfer. The law in every state bars someone who is incompetent from making a legal transfer. If a person can't understand the significance of what he or she is doing, he or she won't be permitted to give away assets.

Example 32

Your father suffers a stroke and becomes incapacitated. As a result, he must be admitted to a nursing home.

Since he is incompetent, he can't transfer his bank accounts, CDs, and stocks. Within a short time, his life savings are gone.

If a person is occasionally competent, he or she can create a valid durable power of attorney during a "lucid moment." In a situation like this, several independent witnesses need to be present when the person signs a durable power of attorney so there can be no question of his or her competence at that time.

A nursing-home resident's spouse cannot transfer the assets because he or she is the spouse; the same holds true for children. No person can act for a nursing-home patient to transfer assets in his or her name just because that person is related.

When someone has become incapacitated and can't handle his or her own affairs, how then is a transfer usually handled? There are two primary vehicles: a guardianship or a durable power of attorney. A guardianship is worthless for Medicaid purposes; a durable power of attorney can be invaluable.

What Is a Guardianship?

A guardian (sometimes known as a conservator, curator, committee, tutor, or fiduciary) can be appointed by a probate court judge for someone who cannot conduct his or her own affairs. Once appointed, a guardian may take any necessary steps, under the probate court's supervision, to manage the finances of the person for whom the guardian is appointed. The guardian must act for the benefit of that person and must report regularly to the probate court.

Could a guardian appointed for your parent transfer his or her assets after your parent enters a nursing home, so that your parent would qualify for Medicaid? After all, isn't that what your parent would do if he or she were competent?

To my knowledge, no judge has ever allowed a guardian to get rid of someone's assets in order to qualify that person for Medicaid. The reason is simple: a person's guardian must watch out for his or her best interests, not the best interests of his or her family; a judge is not likely to say that it's in a person's best interest to become impoverished. In addition, establishing a guardianship is emotionally and financially costly. To have a loved one labeled "incompetent" can be devastating for the family. And the costs generally run at least $2,000 and often much higher.

A less common alternative, appointment of a representative payee, has the same limitations. A representative payee may be appointed under certain public programs (i.e., Social Security or veterans' programs) to receive and spend benefits on behalf of a beneficiary who is unable to manage his or her benefits alone. Again, an elderly person's representative payee can make expenditures only in the best interest of that person and probably will not be permitted to transfer assets from a nursing-home patient in order to qualify the patient for Medicaid.

The only way an older person can avoid appointment of a guardian (or representative payee) should he or she become incompetent is to plan ahead and give someone a durable power of attorney while still able to do so.

What Is a Durable Power of Attorney?

Let's start by talking about a regular power of attorney, because you may already be familiar with that. A regular power of attorney authorizes someone else to act for the maker of the document. The maker is often called the "principal"; the person authorized to act for the principal is called an "attorney-in-fact" or an "agent."

A regular power of attorney can give someone very specific, limited powers. For example, it can authorize someone to sign the deed to sell your house while you are out of town. Or a power of attorney can give someone very broad authority. For example, it may authorize someone to do anything you could do—endorse checks, pay bills, or have access to bank accounts.

A *durable* power of attorney is almost exactly the same as a regular power of attorney, but with one key difference. A *regular* power of attorney becomes ineffective and stops working the moment the maker becomes incompetent; a *durable* power of attorney remains valid even after the maker becomes incompetent.

Since the time an individual may really need a power of attorney is when he or she becomes incompetent, this is no small difference. An older person should have a *durable* power of attorney for his or her protection.

Example 33

Your widowed father suffers a stroke and becomes incapacitated. As a result, he is admitted to a nursing home.

He is incompetent and can't transfer his own assets. But he did give you a durable power of attorney authorizing you to transfer assets. You use that durable power of attorney to transfer assets from your father to you and perhaps among any brothers and/or sisters.

Two and one-half years later, your father's nursing-home tab can be covered by Medicaid, and the rest of his assets will be protected. If at a later date his condition improves and he's able to leave the nursing home, his assets can be transferred back to him.

A durable power of attorney is also crucial to the planning techniques discussed in Chapter 5. For example, I discussed how a nursing-home parent can protect assets by transferring them to his or her children through a spouse-at-home. Since this technique works only if the transfers are made after the parent enters a nursing home, there exists a substantial risk that he or she will not be competent at that time. The success of this technique will depend on whether the parent previously gave the spouse-at-home (or someone else) a durable power of attorney, so that person would then be authorized to make the transfer.

Example 34

Your father is suddenly incapacitated by a stroke and becomes incompetent. Your mother has no choice but to admit him to a nursing home. Since your father is incompetent, he can't transfer the bank accounts, CDs, and stocks in his name. Your mother dies shortly after that, and all but $2,000 of your father's savings will be turned over to the nursing home.

Had your father given your mother a durable power of attorney, she could have used it to transfer assets from your father into her name and/or the names of their children. Then when she died, the financial disaster described in this example would have been averted.

If a person becomes incompetent and has *not* given anyone a durable power of attorney, his or her financial affairs will be carried on by a guardian appointed by the court. And the incompetent person probably will then lose his or her savings to a nursing home.

Can a Person Prepare His or Her Own Durable Power of Attorney?

The answer is yes. A durable power of attorney does not have to be complicated. It must be in writing, signed by the principal, and it must state the name of the person who is being authorized to act for the principal and the scope of his or her powers.

Every state has its own rules governing the use of a durable power of attorney. For example, Florida requires that the attorney-in-fact (the agent named in the durable power of attorney to handle the principal's affairs) be a spouse, parent, adult child, sibling, niece, or nephew of the person making a durable power of attorney. Other important variations are listed in Table 16. Because laws differ significantly concerning use, execution, and recording of durable powers of attorney, and because the

laws are constantly changing, it is always good procedure to check with a lawyer.

At the back of the book, in Appendix A, you will find a facsimile form for your state of residence. Still, because a durable power of attorney is so important, and because state laws can change at any time, it would be best to have an attorney check over your completed form. An attorney's review is a minimal investment, usually $25 to $50, that can assure you as to the authority and correctness of your durable power of attorney, a very important document.

How to Avoid Abuse by the Holder of a Durable Power of Attorney

When you draw up a durable power of attorney, you are giving someone else the right to go into bank accounts, cash checks, sell stocks, and do anything you could do with respect to your own finances. If that makes you uncomfortable, it should!

As soon as you give someone a durable power of attorney, that person can use it—the durable power of attorney is effective immediately, not just when you become incapacitated.

Legally, the person to whom you give a durable power of attorney is limited—he or she can act only in your best interests. If he or she decides to sell your car or house, you are entitled to the money; he or she can't legally raid your accounts and take the money to Tahiti. But as a practical matter, if someone does abuse your trust and misuse the durable power of attorney, you will have a legal nightmare.

Here are four options that can minimize your risks:

- Give a durable power of attorney only to someone who is trustworthy.
- Give it to a third party to hold until it must be used.
- Make a "springing" durable power of attorney.
- Name more than one person in the durable power of attorney.

GIVE A DURABLE POWER OF ATTORNEY ONLY TO SOMEONE YOU TRUST

You shouldn't give just anyone a durable power of attorney. *You should give this document only to a trustworthy individual.* Normally, this means your spouse, a child, or a very close friend.

TABLE 16

**Special Requirements for Creating Durable
Powers of Attorney**

STATE	NOTARY REQUIRED	FILING REQUIRED	OTHER
Arkansas	Yes (or approved by probate court)	Probate court	
California	Yes (or signed by two witnesses)		Attorney-in-fact must be state resident; and if patient is in nursing home, one witness must be patient advocate or ombudsman
Connecticut	Yes		Requires two witnesses
District of Columbia			Real estate may not be transferred through a durable power of attorney
Florida			Only a spouse, parent, adult child, sibling, niece, or nephew may be appointed as attorney-in-fact
Minnesota	Yes		
Missouri	Yes	Recorder of Deeds	
New York	Yes		
North Carolina	Yes	Register of Deeds (copy with clerk of superior court)	
Rhode Island			At least one witness must not be related by blood, marriage, or adoption and must not be entitled to any part of the maker's estate
South Carolina	Yes	Register of Mesne Conveyances	Requires three witnesses
Wyoming		Clerk of District Court (copy with clerk of county court where principal resides)	Must be approved by judge of state district court

SOURCE: Adapted from Table 1: "Durable Powers of Attorney," printed in *Financial Abuse: Prevention and Remedies,* prepared by A. Stephen Hill, Ph.D., December 1987, for the American Association of Retired Persons Public Policy Institute and Legal Counsel for the Elderly; and from Table 6: "Special Requirements for Creating Durable Powers of Attorney," printed in *A Matter of Choice: Planning Ahead for Health Care Decisions,* a publication of the American Association of Retired Persons, prepared for use by U.S. Senators John Heinz and John Glenn. © 1987, American Association of Retired Persons. Reprinted with permission.

The person to whom you give a durable power of attorney does not, in most states, have to live in the same state. But for convenience and speed of action, it is always better to give it to someone who lives reasonably close by.

Although the person you choose is called an "attorney-in-fact," he or she does not have to be a lawyer; the attorney-in-fact also need not be a financial planner, businessperson, accountant, or in any other particular profession. Sure, it's helpful if the recipient of a durable power of attorney has some understanding of finances and the legal impact of a durable power of attorney, but it's not required. The only requirement is that you trust the person to whom you give a durable power of attorney.

GIVE IT TO A THIRD PARTY TO HOLD

Another way to reduce the risks is to give the durable power of attorney to a third person to hold until you need it. For example, you may name your son in the durable power of attorney, and then hand it to a third party, say a friend or lawyer, to hold, with instructions not to give it to your son until you become incapacitated and are unable to handle your own affairs. Only then will your son have access to and be able to use the durable power of attorney.

MAKE A SPRINGING DURABLE POWER OF ATTORNEY

In some states, a durable power of attorney can be written so that it doesn't become effective until you become incapacitated—at that time it "springs" into effect. However, this type of power of attorney has not been accepted in many states yet, and even where it is used, it often invites legal problems over when the maker becomes incapacitated.

NAME MORE THAN ONE PERSON IN THE DURABLE POWER OF ATTORNEY

You may choose to give a single durable power of attorney jointly to two people. The durable power of attorney forms provided in this book will allow you to do this. The benefit of naming two people in one document is that both would have to agree before acting on your behalf. That gives you an added degree of protection—one person can't steal you blind.

But naming two people in the same durable power of attorney may also create problems. Sometimes actions must be taken quickly under a durable power of attorney. Delays will be more likely if two people must act together.

Although there are risks involved in making a durable power of attorney, the benefits *far* outweigh the risks. And if you follow these tips, you can minimize the dangers involved.

Can You Give a Durable Power of Attorney to More Than One Person?

You can give separate durable powers of attorney to as many people as you like. You could give one to each of your three kids, one to Aunt Macey, and one to your lawyer. But I don't advise it.

As I've said, these are powerful documents. If it's risky giving a durable power of attorney to one person, it's more risky to give two or three people durable powers of attorney. Each person you give one to has full powers to act for you.

There are very few occasions when I'd recommend giving out more than one durable power of attorney. In the case of elderly parents both getting up in years, each may want to give one durable power of attorney to the other and another durable power of attorney to a child (so that there will be a greater chance that at least the child will be available should both parents become incapacitated or either die). If you have two children and don't want to show favoritism, you may want to give each child a durable power of attorney. Still, you are best off minimizing the number of durable powers of attorney that you hand around.

Can You Cancel a Durable Power of Attorney?

You can easily cancel a durable power of attorney—in theory—just by declaring that it's canceled. You generally don't even have to put the cancellation in writing; all you need do is announce it to the holder, preferably in the presence of witnesses.

In practice, however, effectively canceling a durable power of attorney may be much harder.

Let's say that you announce that a durable power of attorney you granted to a friend is canceled. Your friend immediately goes to the bank with his durable power of attorney and tries to take out your savings.

The bank personnel won't know that you have canceled the power of attorney; they'll see a document that looks valid, and your friend (some friend!) can take the money and run.

In practice, you would have to try to get back all copies of the durable powers of attorney. But that's not easy, since the friend could have made copies you don't even know about.

Of course you could also give notice of the cancellation, in writing, not only to the holder but also to all those people and institutions (like your bank) whom you believe might be asked to honor the durable power of attorney. But it's usually impossible to predict everyone who may be asked to take some action based upon a durable power of attorney.

If worse comes to worse, you could go to court and have a judge order that all copies be returned. But that's a hassle and expense you don't need. Better to minimize the risk in the first place by giving a durable power of attorney only to someone you trust.

CHAPTER 7 SUMMARY CHECKLIST

Everyone, regardless of age—*right now*—needs a durable power of attorney. A durable power of attorney is the most important tool one can have to accomplish the planning strategies presented throughout this book. You should:

- ✔ Prepare a durable power of attorney for your spouse.

- ✔ Prepare durable powers of attorney for one or more of your children.

- ✔ Give the durable powers of attorney to a third person to hold until it becomes necessary for them to be used.

- ✔ Tell your children who is holding the durable powers of attorney and/or where those documents are located.

8 | How to Use a Medicaid Trust to Protect Savings

What Is a Medicaid Trust?

A Medicaid Trust (also called a Medicaid Qualifying Trust) is another planning tool that can help older people protect their assets from the reach of a nursing home. If correctly done, money and property put into a Medicaid Trust will not be depleted to pay the costs of long-term care.

In a nutshell, a trust allows a person to give ownership of property (real estate, personal property, or money) to a trustee who will hold and manage the property for the benefit of that person and/or others. A Medicaid Trust is simply a particular type of trust that can be used to help an older person qualify for Medicaid.

Medicaid Trusts are often misunderstood. Even many lawyers who don't regularly work with planning for older Americans don't understand these trusts and how they work. But there's really no reason for the mystery.

A trust agreement is just a contract between one party (the "settlor") and another (the "trustee"). As long as an older person (settlor) meets the legal requirements of a Medicaid Trust, what that person puts into a Medicaid Trust contract is basically up to the individual. An older person chooses his or her trustee, who will manage and distribute the trust assets just as that trustee is told to do in the trust contract.

If you decide to set up a Medicaid trust, you can choose how much of your money and property to put into it; you can put all or only a portion of your assets under the control of a Medicaid Trust. At the time you set up a Medicaid Trust, and at any time after it is initially established, you can put assets into the trust simply by signing title over to the trustee.

The types of assets that can be put into a trust are almost unlimited. Clearly cash, CDs, stocks, bonds, and other liquid assets can be put into the trust. Even your house, car, bedroom furniture, jewelry, and household goods can be included.

You *must give up control of the assets* you put into a Medicaid Trust; if you do not satisfy this requirement, the trust won't help for Medicaid qualification. You may still retain the right to the income produced by those assets, and you can provide that, upon your death (and the death of your spouse if you are married), the assets will go to any children you have or any other beneficiary you name.

The primary benefit of a Medicaid Trust is that it can protect assets from a nursing home. Transferring assets into a Medicaid Trust is like giving gifts to another person—assets you put into a Medicaid Trust are no longer yours, so Medicaid can't force you to sell them or give them to a nursing home before it will start paying your nursing-home bills. If you recover enough to return home, your assets would still be intact and the income from them would be available for you to live on. And when you die, the savings you intended to go to your children or other heirs will still be there.

Transfers to a Medicaid Trust must satisfy the asset-transfer rules and generally must be made at least two and one-half years before a person enters a nursing home. Transfers made within that time can render one ineligible for Medicaid for a period.

Here's an example of how a Medicaid Trust can help protect one's nest egg and income.

Example 35

An elderly man's assets, excluding his house, consist of $150,000 in CDs invested at 8 percent/year. He puts that entire amount into a Medicaid Trust, giving up complete control of the assets.

He doesn't need the principal to live on, but he does need the $12,000 annual income generated by the investment. So he provides in the Medicaid Trust contract that he is to receive the income from the trust during his lifetime, and on his death his children will receive the principal in the trust.

Then illness strikes, and he is confined to a nursing home, which charges $25,000 a year. Who pays the bill?

The income from the Medicaid Trust will be paid to the nursing home—but that's only $12,000 (less any allowances, described in Chapter 3, for which he is eligible). The remaining $13,000 annual balance will be picked up by Medicaid.

If he becomes healthy enough to leave the nursing home, the assets he put into the Medicaid Trust will still be there, and the $12,000 annual income will still be available for him to live on. And when he dies, his estate will be distributed according to his wishes, not the nursing home's.

Without a Medicaid Trust, he would have to pay the $13,000 annual balance, and his nest egg would quickly disappear. If he recovered so that he could return home, he would face a life of poverty.

What Benefits Does a Medicaid Trust Provide?

While a Medicaid Trust will help protect one's assets from a nursing home, it offers a number of other benefits too. A Medicaid Trust:

- Helps avoid probate.
- Can help manage assets.
- Lets a parent keep a child's inheritance from him or her until an appropriate age.
- Enables a person to maintain financial privacy when he or she dies.

AVOID PROBATE

Everyone wants to avoid probate. Maybe you've heard about someone who went through a probate that took months and months, and in the end the lawyer obtained more money from the estate than did the heirs. Maybe you have lived through a nightmare like this yourself.

More than twenty years ago, Norman Dacey wrote a book entitled *How to Avoid Probate*, which quickly became a number-one best-seller. In his book, Dacey explained how probate was "victimizing the country's widows and orphans." What is this terrible event at the end of life called probate?

When a person dies, with or without a will, his or her estate normally must be probated. Under the supervision of a probate court, the deceased's money and property must be identified and gathered, all debts must be paid, and the remaining assets must be distributed to those entitled to them.

All this can be time-consuming and expensive. It usually takes at least six months to two years to complete the probate process, *and that's if nothing goes wrong!* I can't tell you how many stories I've heard about probates going on, and on, and on, and on. . . . In the meantime, the deceased's beneficiaries may have to wait to receive their inheritance.

Probate costs vary quite a bit. The primary expenses are the payments to (1) the executor/executrix or administrator/administratrix (the person named in the deceased's will or, if there is no will, a person appointed by the court to manage the distribution of the deceased's estate), and (2) the lawyer for the estate. As a rough rule of thumb, figure probate costs will be at least 2 percent of the value of the estate. They may run as high as 8 to 10 percent of the estate. So for a $150,000 estate, probate costs are likely to range from $3,000 to $15,000—and that's if everything goes smoothly.

What does all this have to do with a Medicaid Trust? Plenty! Any money or property a person puts into a Medicaid Trust will pass to his or her heirs when he or she dies *under the trust*, not under a will, and so will *avoid probate*. A Medicaid Trust takes precedence over a will; money and property in a Medicaid Trust will be distributed upon the settlor's death under the terms of the trust, not under those of the will.

The benefits to a person's heirs may be significant. Such beneficiaries can get their assets immediately under the trust, without the long delays normally involved in probate. And, more important, there are no additional costs, like those involved in probate.

MANAGE ASSETS

Do you need help paying bills, doing banking, or managing investments? Or are you just tired of these chores and looking for relief? A Medicaid Trust may solve such problems.

With a Medicaid Trust, the trustee will help manage your assets. You can have the trustee do everything from pay the mortgage and utilities to balance the checkbook.

More important, a Medicaid Trust can help an older person's spouse or child manage an inheritance after the person has died. For example, let's say that one of your children, though an adult, is a poor financial planner; or maybe the child is disabled and will not be able to handle his or her finances after you're gone. In situations like these, a Medicaid Trust may be the right solution.

You can set up a Medicaid Trust so that it remains in place after you die; instead of distributing assets immediately to a spouse or child, the trustee may continue to manage them for the benefit of the spouse or child during his or her lifetime, just as the trustee did for you while you were alive.

WITHHOLD INHERITANCE

Although none of us plans to die young, unfortunately it sometimes happens. If a person dies leaving young children, someone will have to manage the children's share of their parent's estate.

Most of us appoint a guardian or custodian for minor children in our wills. A guardian or custodian is authorized to manage the children's finances for their benefit.

But a guardian or custodian generally can control children's inheritances only until they reach the age of majority (typically eighteen or twenty-one). At that time, your children will have absolute discretion over how to spend their inheritances and could spend the money on, say, horse-betting, instead of on a college education as you may have intended.

Also, a guardian or custodian must run to court (or, more likely, hire a lawyer to go to court) periodically to report to a probate judge on how he or she is spending the children's money. That itself costs money, which comes out of the children's inheritance. A Medicaid Trust can help avoid those costs.

By leaving your estate in trust for your children, you can have the trustee continue to manage the children's finances. You can decide the appropriate age for your children to receive their inheritances; you may, for instance, choose to keep the money out of your children's hands until they reach twenty-five, thirty, even fifty, if you think that's best. And a trustee does not have to report regularly to the court like a guardian or custodian usually does, so you save your estate that money.

ENSURE PRIVACY

Property going through probate becomes a matter of public record. Nosy neighbors, con artists, and anyone else who wants to know your business can read the will and other papers prepared during the probate process detailing all your money, property, and bills. In other words, your life becomes an open book for anyone who cares to read it.

That may not appeal to you. A Medicaid Trust maintains your privacy. When you die, your assets pass to beneficiaries under the trust, which is *not* public record. No one gets to know your family's affairs.

Are There Drawbacks to a Medicaid Trust?

The answer is yes—although a Medicaid Trust can protect a person's savings from the reach of a nursing home, it is not the right planning tool for many older Americans. There are some *very serious* drawbacks, which include the following:

- You lose control over, and access to, Medicaid Trust assets.
- You must limit your income.
- You will have to keep Medicaid Trust assets and personal assets separate.
- There may be tax considerations.

Each of these is discussed below.

YOU LOSE CONTROL OVER, AND ACCESS TO, MEDICAID TRUST ASSETS

The key to a Medicaid Trust is that you must *give up complete control* over any assets put into the trust. Although you can use the trust agreement to spell out how you want the trustee to handle your estate, you must give up day-to-day control over any assets in the trust. Otherwise, Medicaid will disregard the Medicaid Trust and refuse to pay the bills for your nursing-home care.

A Medicaid Trust must also be *irrevocable* and *unchangeable*. Once you have set up the trust, you can't undo it or change it. You can always add assets to the trust, but you can't remove assets.

Your spouse cannot serve as your trustee. Medicaid would then claim that you have too much control over the assets. Instead, a more distant family member (possibly a child) or an institution (such as a bank) should be appointed trustee.

Your Medicaid Trust will be closely examined by Medicaid bureaucrats. If you have kept any control over your assets in the Medicaid Trust, they'll disregard the trust and have you foot your nursing-home bill.

YOU MUST LIMIT YOUR INCOME

You will have to limit your income to an amount less than the nursing-home costs, or you will lose the primary benefit that a Medicaid Trust provides.

Example 36

Your assets consist of stocks and bonds valued at $250,000 and yielding $25,000 interest and dividends/year. Your Medicaid Trust provides that you get the income.

Should you have to go into a nursing home with an annual bill of $25,000, all your income would go to cover the costs. Medicaid would pay nothing.

Compare Examples 35 and 36. In Example 35, the Medicaid Trust allows the man to protect assets while Medicaid picks up part of the nursing-home costs. In Example 36, the Medicaid Trust makes little sense; you end up paying the entire nursing-home bill.

In other words, if your income is high enough to pay the nursing-home costs, you should either limit the income paid out (plowing the rest back into the Medicaid Trust, or paying it to someone else) or forget about using a trust.

YOU SHOULD KEEP MEDICAID TRUST ASSETS AND PERSONAL ASSETS SEPARATE

You may choose not to place all your assets into a Medicaid Trust. Most people keep at least a small checking account open in their own name.

You will have to keep track of which assets are in the Medicaid Trust and which are not. While this is usually not a major problem, it can be an inconvenience.

THERE MAY BE TAX CONSIDERATIONS

Setting up a Medicaid Trust shouldn't increase or reduce the amount of your income tax. You will still be taxed at the rate you would pay if there were no trust.

A Medicaid Trust also shouldn't add to your state inheritance tax and could possibly decrease it (although a marital deduction, discussed in Chapter 5, won't be available). If your estate is over $600,000, you should consider different types of trusts that can save your estate federal inheritance taxes. Particularly at this higher level of assets, you should consult an experienced tax lawyer for advice; the subject is beyond the scope of this book.

How Much Does a Medicaid Trust Cost?

There are two principal costs:

- Set-up fee
- Management fee

Laws governing Medicaid Trusts vary from state to state. If you decide to use a Medicaid Trust, you should contact a local attorney experienced in Medicaid planning and trust drafting. (See Chapter 12 on the selection of a lawyer.) Unfortunately, as we all know, lawyers don't work for free. A lawyer will charge anywhere between $500 and $2,000 to prepare a simple Medicaid Trust contract. This book provides five simple Medicaid Trust agreement forms—see Appendix B—that can be adapted by a lawyer to fit your specific needs and the requirements of your state law. If you fill out one of the forms in this book and bring it to an attorney, you should be able to reduce the lawyer's fee significantly because the bulk (if not all) of the information needed will already be compiled.

Banks don't work for free either. If you name a bank or some other professional to serve as trustee to manage your funds, you can expect to be charged ³/₄ percent to 1 percent of the trust assets each year. With a $200,000 estate, that means you would pay $1,500 to $2,000 annually.

If you appoint a reliable relative or friend as trustee, you can save these trustee fees.

When Is a Medicaid Trust Useful?

Given the drawbacks and costs of a Medicaid Trust, you may be wondering when a Medicaid Trust should be used. The answer, of course, depends on the circumstances involved.

As discussed in Chapter 7, creation and use of a durable power of attorney can ensure that you contribute no more than about $60,000 (two and one-half years of nursing-home costs). And since use of a durable power of attorney is less drastic than use of a Medicaid Trust, that is often a preferable planning tool.

However, use of a durable power of attorney will require transferring assets to children or others, which could jeopardize your financial security. A Medicaid Trust is probably most useful for people who are concerned about this risk. Consider this example:

Example 37

> Your assets total $100,000. While at home, you need the income from those assets to pay your daily living expenses.
>
> Then you enter a nursing home. Your son uses your durable power of attorney to transfer all of your assets to himself. Six months later, you are able to leave the nursing home and return home. But all of your assets are gone; your son has used them for his own needs. Your main source of income has disappeared.

With a Medicaid Trust, you can be assured that your assets will not be touched during your lifetime and that the income stream from those assets will remain available. If you are worried about a night-

mare like that described in the above example, you may find a Medicaid Trust to be appealing.

The amount of income you receive may also affect the utility of a Medicaid Trust. If you have $300,000 invested at 8 percent, you will be receiving more than enough income to pay the nursing-home bills—whether or not the assets are placed in trust. Only if your income were less than the nursing-home costs, or if you were willing to limit irrevocably your income from assets that would be placed in a Medicaid Trust, would a Medicaid trust be worth considering.

If your income is less than the nursing-home costs *and* you are concerned about giving up your assets to children or others who might dissipate those assets during your nursing-home stay, you should give serious consideration to a Medicaid Trust.

Who Should Be the Trustee?

Under a Medicaid Trust, you are giving up control of your assets to a trustee. Obviously, it's crucial that you select the best possible person to serve.

Your trustee will either be an individual, typically a close relative or friend, or an institution, typically a local bank. Here are guidelines for choosing either type of trustee.

INDIVIDUAL TRUSTEE

These five questions should be considered when selecting a trustee:

Do I trust the person? This is the most important consideration. You are giving a trustee a great deal of power over, and responsibility for, your well-being. Choose someone who will not abuse that power.

Where does the person live? There is no legal requirement that a trustee live in the same state. But you will be *much* better off with a trustee who lives nearby. Convenience is important. For example, you may need quick action by the trustee, and waiting for bills and checks to pass through the mails can prove to be costly.

Is the person willing to accept the job? You should not just name a trustee without first making sure he or she will accept the responsibility. Serving as a trustee can be a lot of work, and your choice may decline the "privilege" of serving, especially if there is no compensation.

Can the person handle the job? If your entire estate is simply savings accounts and CDs, the trustee does not need to be a financial wizard. But if your estate is more complicated, maybe consisting of stocks and bonds that must be sold and bought, real estate that must be managed, or a small business that must be run, it would be wise to select a trustee with the necessary business, financial, or legal experience necessary to handle such affairs.

Is the person a beneficiary of the trust? If you choose to appoint as a trustee someone who will or could be a beneficiary of the trust, there would potentially be some adverse tax consequences to the trustee in situations where the trustee will be making distributions (income and/or principal) of more than $10,000/year. In those situations, the trustee might be considered to be making personal gifts that would be subject to gift-tax laws. If your choice for trustee will or could be a trust beneficiary, you should ask a lawyer about the possible gift-tax implications.

PROFESSIONAL TRUSTEE

You should shop around at local banks and trust companies and not automatically use the bank that holds your savings account. Although the fact that you have received good service there might be one consideration, bank trust departments generally are completely separate from the rest of the bank; you may receive much different service from the trust department's service personnel and administrators.

When you shop around, you should ask:

- What was the performance of the bank's trust funds over the last five years? ten years?
- What fees will be charged?

NO MATTER WHOM YOU CHOOSE, COMPLETE INSTRUCTIONS SHOULD BE PROVIDED

Although you must give up control over the funds once you put them into a Medicaid Trust, that doesn't mean a trustee has absolute discretion to manage the assets. You can use the trust agreement to spell out in great detail exactly how the estate should be managed, the funds invested, and the assets distributed. The trustee can be left with little

more than ministerial responsibilities to carry out your wishes.

For example, you can spell out for the trustee his, her, or its responsibility for:

Investments. Do you want your funds invested conservatively in T-bills, or would you prefer riskier investments in the stock market? You can specify detailed investment strategies, even specific investments.

Distributions. Do you want to be paid the entire income from investments annually or quarterly? Do you want a fixed dollar allowance that might be less or more than the income generated? You can specify exactly how disbursements should be made.

Reporting and Record Keeping. Just because you won't be involved in the daily financial activities doesn't mean the trustee can't provide information about actions taken. You can require that the trustee undertake particular reporting and record-keeping activities.

Management. You may want to give the trustee authority to manage real estate or a business, to buy and sell property, and/or to undertake other specific management responsibilities. All this could be spelled out in the trust agreement.

Tax Returns. Your trustee will have to prepare and file annual tax returns covering the trust activity. Make sure these responsibilities are covered in the trust agreement.

If the trustee is a professional trustee (usually an institution), you may not want to define the investment responsibilities too narrowly. Assuming the trustee has experience and a good track record in managing funds, why mess with success? After all, you are paying the trustee—let the bank earn its keep by making the investments.

Is a Medicaid Trust the Same as a Living Trust?

Don't confuse Medicaid Trusts with other, more common trusts. Two of the most common trusts, living trusts and testamentary trusts, are different in crucial respects from Medicaid Trusts.

The term "living trust" applies literally to any

trust made during a person's lifetime, which theoretically would include a Medicaid Trust. But when you hear the term "living trust," it generally refers to a trust that is freely *revocable and changeable*—if you change your mind about something in a living trust, you can just redo it. A living trust generally is limited to a trust that allows the maker almost complete control over his or her assets. A Medicaid Trust is *very* different.

A testamentary trust also differs significantly from a Medicaid Trust. It generally is created in a person's will and does not take effect until the maker dies. For example, you may want direct control over your money and property during your lifetime, without bothering with a trust; when you die, you will want a trust to help your spouse or children manage the funds. In that case, you might want a testamentary trust.

Since a testamentary trust does not take effect until death, generally it cannot help protect assets from a nursing home. (In limited circumstances, a testamentary trust could be used to protect a couple's assets in case one spouse dies leaving a testamentary trust and the surviving spouse subsequently enters a nursing home.) A testamentary trust doesn't even have the benefit of avoiding probate, since your estate passes under your will (and through probate) into the trust.

Only a Medicaid Trust, meeting all the restrictions described above, can help you protect your assets from the nursing home.

At the back of this book, in Appendix B, are presented five model Medicaid Trusts, one of which may be appropriate to your circumstances or those of your parent or spouse. *By using any of these forms (printed on legal-size sheets in this book), you can save yourself from $500 to more than $1,000 in the costs of having an attorney prepare it for you.* Still, as with the forms for a durable power of attorney (Appendix A), you should have a lawyer check over your completed Medicaid Trust form to make sure it satisfies your needs and current state laws.

CHAPTER 8 SUMMARY CHECKLIST

You can use a Medicaid Trust to protect assets from the catastrophic costs of long-term care, especially if:

- ✔ You have liquid assets (like cash and CDs, but not including a house) of less than about $250,000.

- ✔ You have income of less than $25,000/year or are willing to limit your income to an amount less than $25,000/year.

- ✔ It is not practical for you to transfer all of your money into exempt assets, like a house.

- ✔ You have no child or other loved one to whom you can transfer assets with the expectation that the person will use the assets to care for you, or you just do not want to transfer assets to your children or others.

- ✔ You have not yet entered a nursing home.

- ✔ You want to be sure that income from your assets will be available if you were eventually to return from a nursing home.

9 | As a Last Resort, Get a Divorce

An older couple may be blissfully happy. But if they want to look out for their best interests, they may need to get divorced!

A Divorce Can Protect a Couple's Assets

The new Medicaid Catastrophic Coverage Act has been labeled by some experts as the Divorce Encouragement Law of 1988. That's because, under this new law, if an older couple wants to get around the $60,000 asset ceiling for a spouse-at-home, divorce may be the best way for them to protect their combined nest egg.

Example 38

Your mother and father have combined assets (excluding their home) of $200,000. They split the assets in half, putting $100,000 in your father's name and $100,000 in your mother's name. Then your father enters a nursing home.

Before the Medicaid Catastrophic Coverage Act was passed, the situation described here would have been a very sensible planning approach, "equalizing" assets between spouses. Then when one spouse entered a nursing home, only assets in that spouse's name would be spent on nursing care; the spouse-at-home would conserve his or her half—$100,000—for living expenses.

And your parents actually could have protected more for the spouse-at-home. As soon as your father became ill, all of his assets could have

been transferred to your mother. Even if that transfer didn't occur until the day your father entered a nursing home, he would have been ineligible for Medicaid only for about two years. After spending his funds (about $50,000) for that period of ineligibility, your father would have qualified for Medicaid, and your mother would have salvaged the rest ($150,000) of their combined assets.

Today, your parents couldn't save any more than $62,000.

Example 39

Your mother and father have combined assets of $200,000. Then your father enters a nursing home.

Regardless of whose name the assets are in, the Catastrophic Coverage law allows your mother only the maximum $60,000 and your father $2,000; the remaining $138,000 must be spent on the nursing home before Medicaid begins to pay.

Facing the prospects of poverty, spouses now may have no alternative but divorce.

Example 40

A couple has been married for forty years. They have combined assets of $200,000. The husband is extremely ill and will probably have to enter a nursing home.

The couple files for an uncontested divorce, and the judge grants it. As is usual in divorces, the judge must split the marital property. He awards the husband one-half, $100,000, and the wife the other half. The husband's $100,000 will be paid to the nursing home, but the wife's portion is protected.

Compare Examples 39 and 40—a divorce would have saved your parents $38,000! Although a divorce is certainly a drastic step, especially after a long and happy marriage, the savings to a family's assets can be tremendous.

Not all divorce judges will split the assets evenly under these circumstances. In some cases, a judge may award a larger portion to the spouse who is ill, feeling that he or she needs more owing to higher medical and nursing-care expenses. But more often, divorce judges tilt toward the spouse-at-home, recognizing that the institutionalized spouse will have Medicaid available. Chances are good that the spouse-at-home may be awarded even more than one-half of the couple's combined assets in a divorce.

A Divorce Can Protect Income

A divorce can be crucial to protecting *assets*. It usually is much less important to protect *income* for the spouse-at-home, although in some cases it may be helpful here too.

Example 41

A couple is living on the modest amount of $1,575/month: the husband's pension payments of $375 and Social Security benefits of $800; and the wife's Social Security benefits of $400. Then the husband enters a nursing home.

About four years ago, a case with the same facts went before a court in New York. A woman designated in the court papers as Rose Septuagenarian asked the court to grant her support from her institutionalized husband after Medicaid insisted that his entire income, $1,175/month, should be used to pay his nursing costs, leaving Rose to live on just $400/month. Rose was devoted to her husband and regularly visited him at the nursing home; she was seeking reasonable support payments only to allow her to maintain a modest standard of living.

The New York Medicaid officials argued that no support should be allowed. They pointed out that Rose's husband was receiving Medicaid, a form of public assistance, and so could not support himself, let alone his spouse. Her husband's medical and living expenses far exceeded his income, so they argued that all his income should be applied to those expenses before any deduction for Rose's support.

The divorce judge, Jeffrey H. Gallet, disagreed, displaying compassion and uncommon common sense. Judge Gallet said that:

> [T]o deprive women, and particularly women of [Rose's] generation who, in many cases, were denied an equal opportunity to fulfill their potential in the employment market and are, therefore, dependent on their husbands for support, access to their husbands' pension and assets in their later years effectively sentences many of them to tremendous hardship and a complete disruption of their lives at a time when they are extremely vulnerable.
>
> We must note that an overwhelming majority of married women are younger than their husbands. In addition, actuarial tables tell us that women live longer than men . . . (for example, a woman of 70 will outlive her 75-year-old husband by more than 11 years . . .). From those facts, together with the common knowledge that medical costs for many illnesses of old age are beyond the financial means of most American families, we can reasonably draw the conclusion that husbands are more likely to require care which will deplete the marital assets than their wives, who are likely to be the economically weaker spouse. So in cases such as this, where the petitioner is 72 years old and infirm, women will be forced from their homes, deprived of even their modest life-styles and relegated to a life of grinding poverty.

(From the case of *In re Rose Septuagenarian*, 126 Misc. 2d 699, Family Court, Queens County, Judge Jeffrey H. Gallet.)

Judge Gallet ended up awarding Rose support from her husband of $1,125/month; only $50/month was paid to the nursing home, with Medicaid picking up the rest of the tab.

The law has changed since the case of Rose Septuagenarian. Under the recently passed Medicaid Catastrophic Coverage Act, the spouse-at-home may be entitled to an allowance from the nursing-home spouse based on a complicated formula discussed in Chapter 3 (see pages 24–25). Although the amount permitted under the new law can be a hardship, the spouse-at-home won't be left with virtually no income as Rose almost was.

Still, a divorce may enhance the spouse-at-home's income. (In some states, including New York, support can be awarded without a divorce.) Let's look back at Example 4. In that case, the couple was living on a combined income of $3,400/month until the husband entered a nursing home. At that time, under the new law, the wife's income would be reduced to $1,150.20/month ($400 of her own income and $750.20 from her husband). Although she wouldn't starve on $1,150.20, it would still be much less each month than she had had before. A divorce (or support order) might yield a higher income.

Don't Wait Too Long for a Divorce

A divorce can be a very helpful planning tool, especially to protect assets for the spouse-at-home. But there's a hitch—the couple can't wait too long. While divorce should be only the planning tool of last resort, if a couple puts the decision off too long, they may lose the opportunity to take advantage of this technique.

They may not be able to obtain a divorce once the nursing-home spouse becomes incompetent. Many divorce judges are reluctant to grant a divorce from an incompetent spouse. And even if the couple should get a divorce, it would likely be only at great legal and emotional costs.

Once a nursing-home spouse becomes incompetent, the first step is likely to require a trip to probate court before a divorce can proceed. A probate judge will declare your spouse incompetent and name a guardian who will then represent the spouse in the divorce case.

A guardian has a legal duty to act in your incompetent spouse's best interests, which may not be the same as your own best interests, or those of any children you may have. The guardian may even have a legal obligation to oppose the divorce on the grounds that, given your spouse's high medical costs, no assets should be given away—even if Medicaid could pick up those same costs!

In other words, once one spouse becomes incompetent, divorce becomes a much less attractive planning tool. If an elderly couple is considering a divorce as the way to protect their savings, they can't put off the decision too long.

Spouses who find themselves facing tremendous nursing-home costs may *have* to consider a divorce. However unpleasant the prospect for such a happily married couple, the financial devastation resulting from staying together could prove to be even more unpleasant.

10 Private Insurance for Long-Term Care

Many older Americans believe that they don't need to worry very much about the costs of long-term care because they assume Medicare and Medicare supplemental insurance will provide coverage. Wrong! Right now, *no one* is covered for long-term nursing-home care under Medicare or standard Medigap policies, and very few older Americans are covered under any insurance.

This is not to say that there is no insurance available to cover long-term nursing-home costs. A growing number of long-term-care policies are being offered, and if one is willing to do some homework, the right policy may be found at an affordable cost.

Following is a discussion of private insurance options currently available.

Medigap Policies Won't Cover Long-Term-Care Needs

Television personalities like Art Linkletter, Danny Thomas, and Michael Landon have been promoting Medigap insurance policies for the elderly. Many of these ads give the impression that these policies will "fill the gaps" left by an older person's Medicare coverage. Millions of Americans have purchased private supplemental health care coverage thinking that these policies will pay their nursing-home costs.

Unfortunately, many of these Medigap policies are not all they're cracked up to be. Often they won't cover a person's basic health care costs, let alone long-term nursing-home expenses. In fact, many Americans have been duped into purchasing *several* Medigap policies providing duplicate coverage. One Arkansas man told a U.S. House of Representatives subcommittee that his aunt had been sold twenty-eight Medigap policies with the understanding that necessary long-term-care costs would be covered. When she did need help, not one of the policies provided coverage. No matter how many Medigap policies a person buys, they will *not* meet his or her long-term-care needs.

I am not suggesting that Medigap policies are worthless—*one* good policy *may* be a worthwhile investment. Medigap policies supplement Medicare and vary greatly in coverage and eligibility requirements.

But even the best Medigap policies will cover very little of a person's nursing-home costs. As discussed in Chapter 1, Medicare generally pays for part of the costs of a skilled nursing home for the first eight days and all of a resident's costs for the next 142 days; most Medigap policies will pay the difference not paid by Medicare for just those first eight days. Some Medigap policies provide limited *skilled*-care coverage beyond the 150-day Medicare limit, but that helps very few people. *No* Medigap policy provides coverage for custodial (nonskilled) long-term care.

Long-Term Insurance May Be the Answer

A new type of insurance, commonly called long-term-care insurance, is becoming more widely available throughout the country. Today about seventy private insurance companies, including many of the largest such as Prudential, Fireman's Fund, and Aetna, offer long-term-care policies. These policies vary widely as to coverage and cost. So far they have proved of limited utility because of their expense, restrictions, limitations, and eligibility requirements and as a result only about 500,000 policies have been sold.

Still, for some families a well-chosen policy may be a worthwhile alternative to losing their savings to a nursing home, particularly if they are still healthy.

Before even beginning to look for a private long-term-care insurance policy, the older person should check to see if he or she is already covered. Although the chances are extremely slim, it's worth the investment of time. If the person is covered by a group health insurance plan sponsored by an employer, union, trade association, or some other organization, he or she should ask the benefits representative about what benefits are included, particularly after retirement.

Also, it might be worthwhile for the person to check with any health maintenance organizations in the area. Sometimes HMOs offer a good long-term-care package at a more reasonable price than that for long-term-care insurance.

But, most likely, the person will find that he or she is not yet covered and that no HMO offers a reasonable option. Then it will be time to look at long-term-care insurance.

What You Should Look For in a Nursing-Home Policy

Nursing-home policies currently on the market vary greatly in cost and coverage. Here is a twenty-two-point, five-part checklist to use when investigating the available options.

THE COST OF THE POLICY

What Is the Annual Premium?

The major reason long-term-care policies haven't caught fire is the premium—this is generally *expensive* insurance. Premiums vary depending on a number of factors, including the company, the insuree's age and health, the amount and type of benefits provided, and the length of time the insuree has to cover the nursing-home tab himself or herself before

insurance coverage begins (as with a deductible).

Age is the most significant element; the exact same policy may cost a sixty-year-old $100/year, a seventy-year-old $3,000, and an eighty-year-old $10,000 annually.

Premium rates can range widely, from $100 to $10,000/year. Generally, a person will be guaranteed the same premium each year, without its going up over time.

Can the Company Raise the Premium?

You should check to make sure the policy is renewable *at the same rates*. If the rates can be increased, the insuree could be forced to give up his or her policy. Note that even a guaranteed rate may not always remain unchanged. If the insurer increases the premium on a policy for everyone in the state, that will probably be allowed.

WHAT THE POLICY PAYS

How Much Is the Daily Benefit Payment?

Long-term-care insurance, though called insurance, is really an indemnity plan in most cases. Instead of paying some portion of nursing-care bills, these policies generally pay a set daily dollar amount for a specified time while one is in a nursing home—regardless of how high the expenses run.

Most policies let the insuree choose the amount of coverage, usually running from $30 to $120/day for skilled nursing care, less for more typical custodial care (if that's even covered). Of course, the higher the benefit provided, the more costly the premium. You should check the costs for nursing homes in the community—experts recommend that an insuree try to obtain a benefit amount that will cover at least one-half to two-thirds of the average daily cost for nursing homes in his or her area. Any less than that won't be very helpful. If the policy pays $30/day and nursing homes in your area charge $90/day, a lifetime of savings could quickly be depleted.

THE BENEFITS

What Types of Long-Term-Care Expenses Are Covered?

You should check to see if the policy covers skilled, intermediate, custodial, and home care. Any policy should cover *all* these types of care; otherwise the person may discover—after it's too late—that the policy won't pay for the type of care he or she needs.

If nothing else, you should make sure the policy pays for custodial care, which is the type of care most often required. Custodial care covers nursing-home residents who need help with routine daily activities like walking, eating, going to the toilet, and bathing. A policy that covers only skilled care provided by doctors, nurses, and therapists may be of very little use, since few long-term residents need that kind of assistance.

You should also check to see whether the policy limits care to a particular type of facility. For example, the policy might cover skilled, intermediate, and custodial care but only in a skilled nursing-home facility. Again, that limitation could render the policy useless. You should choose a policy that covers custodial care in any nursing-home facility.

A number of policies also offer coverage of services provided at home. These may include nursing, housecleaning, even meal preparation. You should check whether the policy provides home-service coverage, for what period, at what cost, and with what conditions and limitations. While home-service coverage is not absolutely necessary, it may be just the answer for keeping one out of a nursing home altogether.

When Do Benefits Start?

Some policies begin paying benefits the first day a person enters a hospital or nursing home, whereas others wait a certain period, often twenty to one hundred days, before starting benefit payments. Since many nursing-home stays are relatively short, fewer than one hundred days, you should find a policy with a short waiting period—twenty days or less.

How Long Will the Benefits Last?

Benefits are usually paid for one to six years; six years is more than enough to cover most stays, although some policies offer benefits for an unlimited period. Obviously, the longer the term, the more desirable the policy. Check the benefit period for both skilled and custodial care—it may differ for each type of care coverage.

Also check the policy's rules for repeat nursing-home stays. For example, the insurer may require the insuree to have been out of a nursing home for six months before he or she will qualify for benefits on a subsequent stay.

Does the Plan Offer an Inflation-Protection Option?

Long-term-care plans typically pay a fixed daily amount. But whereas such benefits will be fixed, nursing-home costs won't be. Inflation surely will cause costs to rise. A person may not need benefits for ten years, by which time daily rates may be *much higher* than what they are today.

For example, using a conservative 5 percent annual inflation rate, a $70 daily charge in 1988 would be about $81 in 1991 (around $30,000 annually), $109 in 1997 (around $40,000 annually), and $126 in the year 2000 (around $46,000 annually). Only with inflation protection can one be sure his or her policy will provide adequate protection. Unfortunately, only a handful of policies offer such inflation protection. Particularly if an insuree is under sixty, he or she shouldn't consider a policy without this option.

Does the Policy Provide Benefits for Necessary Care While Away from Home or After Moving to Another State?

You should find out whether the coverage still applies if something happens while one is traveling or if one has moved. Since no one would want to be a prisoner at home, or to lose the policy coverage by moving, this could be an important option.

Does the Policy Contain a Premium-Waiver Option?

Some policies say that, after an insuree has been receiving benefits for a certain period, usually ninety days, he or she doesn't have to continue to pay premiums and the policy will remain in force. This may be an important provision, because once a nursing-home resident has begun an extended stay, he or she may no longer be able to afford premiums.

Is There a Grace Period for Late Payment?

Policies often provide a grace period (typically a week to a month) during which the policy continues even if the insuree is late with the premium. Without any grace period, a policy could be canceled immediately.

Does the Insurer Give the Insuree a "Free Look"?

Many policies allow the insuree to cancel and obtain a full refund within a specified period after he or she signs up—typically ten to thirty days. In fact, most states *require* the insurer to provide this money-back guarantee.

Can the Policy Be Upgraded?

Long-term-care insurance is fairly new on the market, and products are constantly changing. You should look to see if a policy gives the right to switch to a better policy as improvements are made.

LIMITS OF THE POLICY

Does the Policy Contain Health- or Age-Eligibility Requirements?

Most policies impose health- and age-eligibility requirements. Policies typically will exclude applicants who are over a specified age (usually eighty) or who, owing to poor health, may no longer be able to care for themselves.

Just because a person may not be healthy enough to qualify for life or health insurance doesn't mean he or she won't qualify for long-term-care insurance. For example, terminal cancer may disqualify a person for life insurance since his or her life expectancy is short, but that same person could be a good risk for long-term-care insurance.

How Does the Policy Treat Existing Medical Conditions?

Even if one is eligible to buy insurance, policies typically either exclude preexisting conditions or impose a waiting period before coverage goes into effect for those conditions.

Preexisting conditions are generally defined as medical conditions that were diagnosed or treated, or which should have been diagnosed or treated based on their symptoms, prior to purchasing the policy. Insurers typically look back at conditions that existed within six months to three years of the application for coverage; if the condition existed more than three years before application, the applicant shouldn't have trouble obtaining coverage.

Policies that impose a waiting period vary on the length of the period. Waiting periods usually last for three to six months.

Don't ignore health conditions in the policy just because the insurance carrier may not require a medical examination. Insurees are still required to provide accurate information about their health, and if it is later discovered that they were not truthful, they may lose all benefits.

Does the Policy Restrict Coverage by Requiring a Hospital Stay?

Many policies provide that they will pay benefits only if the insuree enters a nursing home after a hospital stay of at least three days. How much time may pass between leaving the hospital and entering a nursing home will vary, with policies typically allowing no more than thirty to ninety days to pass. Since 60 percent of people admitted to nursing homes, including many suffering from Alzheimer's disease or arthritis, were not first in a hospital, this limitation renders the policy worthless for most nursing-home residents.

Does the Policy Require Skilled Nursing Care to Precede Custodial Care?

A requirement that the insuree must first receive skilled care before the policy will cover intermediate or custodial care, like the hospital-stay requirement, can severely limit the usefulness of the policy.

Is a Prior Nursing-Home Stay Required Before the Policy Will Pay for Home Health Care?

Like the two requirements discussed above, the requirement of a prior nursing-home stay may limit the value of the policy.

Are Any Injuries or Diseases Not Covered?

Most policies won't cover mental disorders with a psychological origin. Some insurers use this to refuse coverage of Alzheimer's disease, Parkinson's disease, and senility. You should check any policy closely and make sure that it will cover these three diseases, which land so many older Americans in nursing homes.

You should also look to see whether the policy excludes other injuries or diseases, such as alcoholism and mental retardation.

Is There a Total Dollar Limitation?

The policy may place a dollar limitation on the total lifetime benefit payment that can be made. Obviously, the amount at which this limit is set can affect the value of the policy.

Can the Company Cancel or Refuse to Renew the Policy?

Your policy should be *guaranteed* renewable, which means that its coverage can't be canceled just because the insuree's health has become poor or because of increased age. Under a guaranteed renewable policy, a person can retain coverage as long as he or she pays the premiums.

Also watch out for a policy that is renewable at the option of the insurer; that is not the same as a guaranteed renewable policy. Without a guaranteed renewable policy, an insuree could lose coverage at the very time he or she needs it most.

COMPARING THE COMPANIES

What Is the Insurer's Best Rating?

A. M. Best Company grades the financial stability of insurance companies from A+ (excellent) to C (fair). The lower the rating, the greater the risk that the company won't be around when the insuree needs to obtain the promised benefits.

Does the Insurer Have Local Agents?

Check to see if the insurance company is licensed in the state and has local agents available. That way, if questions have to be asked or something goes wrong, a person will be there to help.

On pages 71–72 is a long-term-care insurance questionnaire based on the above checklist to use for comparing policies.

Recommended Features

When you evaluate long-term-care policies, *Consumer Reports Magazine* (May 1988 article entitled "Who Can Afford a Nursing Home?") recommends that you try to find a policy with these features:

- A daily nursing-home benefit of at least $80
- A waiting period of no more than twenty days

- A benefit period (for one stay) of at least four years
- An unlimited benefit period for all stays
- Benefits provided for skilled, intermediate, custodial, and home care
- If it has a prior-hospitalization rule, coverage beginning no more than thirty days after a hospital stay of three days
- A waiver of premium
- Guaranteed renewable for life
- Specific coverage for Alzheimer's disease
- Guaranteed level premium for life
- A. M. Best Company rating of A or A+

No policy is likely to offer every one, or even most, of these features at a price you can afford. What you must do is look at all factors, decide which are most important in your case, and weigh the benefits against the costs. You pay for quality. The better the coverage, the more the cost.

When checking and comparing policies, do not rely on statements made by salespeople. Sales pitches are often unclear or misleading at best, intentionally false at worst. If you are told that Alzheimer's disease is covered but the policy itself doesn't say that, don't expect the insurer to pay.

It is important to review the policy itself before deciding to buy. If a salesperson refuses to send a policy, you should call the company directly to ask for one. If that request is denied, you have a strong indication that you should look elsewhere.

Companies That Offer Private Long-Term-Care Insurance

In the last few years, the number of companies offering long-term-care insurance policies has grown significantly. Tables 17 and 18 present a sample listing of companies offering long-term-care policies and the states in which such policies were offered at the time of this writing. You might also contact your state insurance department to find out which companies offer long-term-care policies.

The companies in Table 17 are listed in alphabetical order; no ranking is implied. If you want a ranking list, *Consumer Reports* in its May 1988 issue rated fifty-three long-term-care policies, analyzing the same types of factors previously discussed. Reprints may be available by writing to: Reprints, Consumers Union, 256 Washington Street, Mount Vernon, NY 10553.

LONG-TERM-CARE INSURANCE QUESTIONNAIRE

How Much Does the Policy Cost?

1. What is the annual premium?
   $ _____

2. Can the company raise the premium over time or under other circumstances?
   yes _____   no _____
   If so, under what circumstances?
   _____

How Much Does the Policy Pay?

3. What is the maximum amount the policy will pay?
   - skilled nursing care $ _____ per day
   - intermediate nursing care $ _____ per day
   - custodial nursing care $ _____ per day
   - home health care $ _____ per day

What Are the Benefits?

4. What types of long-term care expenses are covered?
   - skilled nursing care   yes _____   no _____
   - intermediate nursing care   yes _____   no _____
   - custodial nursing care   yes _____   no _____
   - home health care   yes _____   no _____

5. When do benefits start?
   - skilled nursing care   _____ days after entering hospital/nursing home
   - intermediate nursing care   _____ days after entering hospital/nursing home
   - custodial nursing care   _____ days after entering hospital/nursing home
   - home health care   _____ days after entering hospital/nursing home
   - all of the above services   _____ days after entering hospital/nursing home

6. How long will the benefits last?
   - skilled nursing care   _____ days
   - intermediate nursing care   _____ days
   - custodial nursing care   _____ days
   - home health care   _____ days
   - all of the above services   _____ days

7. Does the plan offer inflation protection?
   yes _____   no _____

8. Does the policy provide benefits while away from home or after moving to another state?
   yes _____   no _____

9. Does the policy contain a premium-waiver option?
   yes _____   no _____

10. Is there a grace period for late payment?
    yes _____   no _____
    If so: _____ days

11. Does the insurer offer a "free look"?
    yes _____   no _____
    If so: _____ days

12. Can the policy be upgraded?
    yes _____   no _____

What Are the Limits?

13. Does the policy contain health- or age-eligibility requirements?
    yes _____   no _____
    If so, are you eligible for coverage?
    yes _____   no _____

14. a. Does the policy exclude coverage for any conditions you presently have?
       yes _____   no _____
    b. How far back will the company look for preexisting conditions?
       _____ months
    c. Does the company impose a waiting period?
       yes _____   no _____
       If so: _____ months

15. Is a prior hospital stay required before the policy will pay for:
    • skilled care   yes _____   no _____   If so: _____ days
    • intermediate care   yes _____   no _____   If so: _____ days
    • custodial care   yes _____   no _____   If so: _____ days

16. Is a prior skilled nursing-home stay required before the policy will pay for:
    • intermediate care   yes _____   no _____   If so: _____ days
    • custodial care   yes _____   no _____   If so: _____ days

17. Is a prior nursing-home stay required before the policy will pay for:
    • home health care   yes _____   no _____   If so: _____ days

18. Does the policy explicitly cover:
    • Alzheimer's disease   yes _____   no _____
    • Parkinson's disease   yes _____   no _____
    • senility   yes _____   no _____

19. Is there a total dollar limitation?
    yes _____   no _____
    If so: $ _____

20. Can the company cancel or refuse to renew a policy?
    yes _____   no _____
    If there are conditions, what are they:
    _____

How Does the Company Compare to Others?

21. What is the company's Best rating?
    _____

22. Does the company have local agents?
    yes _____   no _____

SOURCE: Adapted from *The Consumer's Guide to Long-Term Care Insurance*, Health Insurance Association of America, 1001 Pennsylvania Avenue, N.W., Washington, D.C. 20004–2599, 1988, reprinted with permission.

TABLE 17

Representative List of Long-Term-Care Health Insurance Carriers (by State)

COMPANY	AL	AK	AZ	AR	CA	CO	CT	DE	DC	FL	GA	HI	ID	IL	IN	IA	KS
Aetna Life and Casualty Co.	X	X	X	X	X	X	X	X		X	X	X	X	X	X		X
AIG Life Insurance Co.	X	X	X	X	X	X	X	X	X	X	X	X	X	X	X	X	X
American Integrity Ins. Co.	X	X	X	X	X	X		X	X	X	X	X	X	X	X	X	X
American Progressive Life & Health Ins. Co. of NY																	
American Republic Ins. Co.	X		X	X	X	X	X	X	X	X	X	X	X	X	X	X	X
Amex Life Assurance Co.	X	X	X	X	X	X	X	X	X	X	X	X	X	X	X	X	X
Bankers Life & Casualty Co.	X	X	X	X	X	X	X	X	X	X	X	X	X	X	X	X	X
Bankers Multiple Line Ins. Co.	X	X	X	X			X	X			X	X	X	X	X	X	X
Central States Health & Life Ins. Co. of Omaha	X	X	X	X	X	X	X	X			X	X	X	X	X	X	X
Certified Life Ins. Co.																	
CNA Insurance Co.	X	X	X	X	X	X		X	X	X	X	X	X	X	X	X	
Colonial Penn Life Ins. Co.	X	X	X	X	X			X	X	X	X	X	X	X	X	X	
Continental American	X	X	X	X	X	X		X			X	X	X	X		X	
Continental General Ins. Co	X	X	X	X	X	X		X			X		X	X	X	X	X
Federal Home Life Ins. Co.													X	X	X	X	X
Fidelity Security Life Ins. Co.		X		X	X	X		X	X	X	X	X	X	X	X	X	X
Gerber Life Ins. Co.																	
John Hancock										X							
Harvest Life Ins. Co.	X	X								X			X				
Mutual of Omaha Ins. Co.	X	X	X	X	X	X	X	X	X	X	X	X	X	X	X	X	X
National States Ins. Co.	X	X		X		X					X		X	X	X	X	
Providers Fidelity Life Ins. Co.	X			X	X	X		X	X	X	X		X	X	X		
Pyramid Life Ins. Co.	X	X	X	X	X	X		X	X	X	X	X		X	X	X	X
Reserve Life Ins. Co.	X		X							X							
Sentry Life Insurance Co.	X	X	X	X	X	X		X	X	X	X	X	X	X	X	X	
Transport Life Ins. Co.	X	X	X	X	X	X		X	X	X	X	X	X	X	X	X	
Union Bankers	X	X	X	X		X		X	X	X	X	X	X	X	X	X	X
Union Fidelity	X	X	X		X	X		X	X	X	X	X	X	X	X	X	
Washington Square Life Ins.	X													X			
World Insurance Co.			X	X		X		X					X				
World Life & Health Ins. Company of PA			X	X				X					X	X			

(continued on next page)

TABLE 17 (continued)

Representative List of Long-Term-Care Health Insurance Carriers (by State)

COMPANY	KY	LA	ME	MD	MA	MI	MN	MS	MO	MT	NE	NV	NH	NJ	NM	NY	NC
Aetna Life and Casualty Co.	X	X	X	X	X	X		X	X	X	X	X	X	X	X	X	X
AIG Life Insurance Co.	X	X		X	X			X	X	X	X	X		X	X	X	
American Integrity Ins. Co.	X	X	X	X	X			X	X	X	X	X		X	X	X	X
American Progressive Life & Health Ins. Co. of NY								X	X	X	X	X		X	X	X	
American Republic Ins. Co.	X							X	X	X	X						X
Amex Life Assurance Co.	X	X	X	X	X	X		X	X	X	X	X	X	X	X		X
Bankers Life & Casualty Co.	X	X	X	X	X	X	X	X	X	X	X	X	X		X		X
Bankers Multiple Line Ins. Co.	X	X		X	X	X	X	X	X	X	X	X	X	X	X		X
Central States Health & Life Ins. Co. of Omaha	X	X	X	X	X	X	X	X	X	X	X	X	X	X	X		X
Certified Life Ins. Co.																	
CNA Insurance Co.	X	X	X	X	X	X	X	X	X	X	X	X	X	X	X		X
Colonial Penn Life Ins. Co.	X	X	X	X	X			X	X	X	X	X	X		X		X
Continental American	X				X			X		X	X			X	X		
Continental General Ins. Co	X	X	X	X		X		X	X	X	X	X			X		
Federal Home Life Ins. Co.																	
Fidelity Security Life Ins. Co.		X	X	X	X	X	X		X	X	X	X	X	X	X		
Gerber Life Ins. Co.																	
John Hancock																X	
Harvest Life Ins. Co.	X	X	X	X	X	X	X	X	X	X	X	X	X	X		X	X
Mutual of Omaha Ins. Co.	X	X		X	X	X	X	X	X	X	X	X	X	X	X	X	
National States Ins. Co.	X	X						X	X	X	X	X			X		
Providers Fidelity Life Ins. Co.	X	X		X	X				X	X	X			X	X		
Pyramid Life Ins. Co.	X								X	X	X						
Reserve Life Ins. Co.						X											
Sentry Life Insurance Co.	X	X	X	X	X	X	X	X	X	X	X	X	X	X	X	X	X
Transport Life Ins. Co.	X	X	X	X	X	X		X	X	X	X	X	X	X	X		X
Union Bankers	X	X	X	X	X			X	X	X	X	X	X		X		X
Union Fidelity	X	X	X		X			X		X	X			X	X		X
Washington Square Life Ins.								X	X			X					
World Insurance Co.	X						X	X	X	X	X						
World Life & Health Ins. Company of PA			X		X		X			X	X				X		

COMPANY	ND	OH	OK	OR	PA	RI	SC	SD	TN	TX	UT	VT	VA	WA	WV	WI	WY
Aetna Life and Casualty Co.		X	X	X	X		X	X	X	X	X	X	X		X		X
AIG Life Insurance Co.	X	X	X				X	X	X	X	X	X		X	X		X
American Integrity Ins. Co.	X	X	X	X	X	X	X	X	X	X	X		X	X	X	X	X
American Progressive Life & Health Ins. Co. of NY					X												
American Republic Ins. Co.	X	X	X	X	X		X	X	X	X	X	X	X	X	X		X
Amex Life Assurance Co.	X	X	X	X	X	X	X	X	X	X	X	X	X	X	X	X	X
Bankers Life & Casualty Co.		X	X	X	X	X	X	X	X	X	X	X	X	X	X	X	X
Bankers Multiple Line Ins. Co.	X	X	X	X	X	X	X	X	X	X	X	X	X	X	X	X	X
Central States Health & Life Ins. Co. of Omaha	X	X	X	X	X	X	X	X	X	X	X	X	X	X	X		X
Certified Life Ins. Co.																	X
CNA Insurance Co.	X	X	X	X	X	X	X	X	X	X	X	X	X	X	X	X	X
Colonial Penn Life Ins. Co.	X	X	X	X	X		X	X	X	X		X	X		X	X	X
Continental American		X	X		X			X			X						X
Continental General Ins. Co		X	X				X	X	X	X	X	X	X	X	X		X
Federal Home Life Ins. Co.				X							X			X			
Fidelity Security Life Ins. Co.	X	X	X		X	X		X	X		X	X	X	X	X		X
Gerber Life Ins. Co.																	
John Hancock		X															
Harvest Life Ins. Co.	X	X	X	X	X		X	X	X	X	X	X	X	X	X		
Mutual of Omaha Ins. Co.	X	X	X	X	X	X	X	X	X	X	X	X	X	X	X	X	X
National States Ins. Co.	X	X	X	X			X	X	X	X	X		X	X	X		
Providers Fidelity Life Ins. Co.	X	X	X	X		X		X	X	X	X		X				X
Pyramid Life Ins. Co.		X	X	X				X	X	X		X	X				
Reserve Life Ins. Co.		X	X					X	X	X							
Sentry Life Insurance Co.	X	X	X		X	X	X	X	X	X		X	X	X		X	X
Transport Life Ins. Co.	X	X	X		X	X	X	X	X	X	X	X	X	X	X	X	X
Union Bankers		X	X	X	X	X		X	X	X	X	X	X		X		
Union Fidelity		X															
Washington Square Life Ins.		X															
World Insurance Co.		X					X	X	X		X	X			X		X
World Life & Health Ins. Company of PA		X		X	X		X				X	X					X

Note: The companies listed all meet the National Association of Insurance Commissioners' Model Act definition of a long-term-care insurance policy. The table does not include all companies selling long-term insurance products.

SOURCE: Health Insurance Association of America. Reprinted with permission.

TABLE 18

Representative List of Long-Term-Care Health Insurance Carriers Home Office Addresses

Aetna Life and Casualty Co.
151 Farmington Avenue
Hartford, CT 06156
516/663-1523

AIG Life Insurance Co.
1 ALICO Plaza
600 King Street
Wilmington, DE 19803
302/594-2000

American Integrity Ins. Co.
Two Penn Center Plaza
Philadelphia, PA 19102-1797
215/561-1400

American Progressive Life & Health
Ins. Co. of NY
P.O. Box 23
Brewster, NY 10509
1-800-243-9214 (outside NY)
1-800-332-3377 (in NY)

American Republic Ins. Co.
P.O. Box 1
Des Moines, IA 50334
1-800-247-2190

AMEX Life Assurance Co.
1650 Los Gamos Road
San Rafael, CA 94903
1-800-231-1133 ext. 582

Bankers Life & Casualty Co.
4444 West Lawrence Avenue
Chicago, IL 60630
312/777-7000 ext. 6120

Bankers Multiple Line Ins. Co.
4444 West Lawrence
Chicago, IL 60630
1-800-572-5189 (in Illinois)
1-800-621-3724 (all states
            except Alaska)

Central States Health & Life Ins.
Co. of Omaha
P.O. Box 34350
Omaha, NE 68134
402/397-1111

Certified Life Ins. Co.
14724 Ventura Boulevard
Sherman Oaks, CA 91403
1-800-258-4400

CNA Ins. Co.
CNA Plaza
Chicago, IL 60685
312/822-5944

Colonial Penn Life Ins. Co.
11 Penn Center Plaza
Philadelphia, PA 19181
1-800-228-5610

Continental American
300 Continental Drive
Wilmington, DE 19885
1-800-441-7004

Continental General Ins. Co.
8901 Indiana Hills Drive
Omaha, NE 68114
402/397-3200

Federal Home Life Ins. Co.
78 West Michigan Avenue
Battle Creek, MI 49017
616-968-7312

Fidelity Security Life Ins. Co.
3130 Broadway
Kansas City, MO 64111
1-800-821-7303 (in Kansas)
1-800-892-7272 (outside Kansas)

Gerber Life Ins. Co.
66 Church Street
White Plains, NY 10601
1-800-253-3155

John Hancock
P.O. Box 111
Boston, MA 02117
1-800-527-4620

Harvest Life Ins. Co.
78 West Michigan Avenue
Battle Creek, MI 49017
616-968-7312

Mutual of Omaha Ins. Co.
Mutual of Omaha Plaza
Omaha, NE 68175
402/342-7600

National States Ins. Co.
11433 Olde Cabin Road
St. Louis, MO 63141
314/997-1191

Providers Fidelity Life Ins. Co.
P.O. Box 1120
Blue Bell, PA 19422-0778
215/542-7200

Pyramid Life Ins. Co.
6201 Johnson Drive
Shawnee Mission, KS 66202
913/722-1110 (call collect)

Reserve Life Ins. Co.
P.O. Box 660254
Dallas, TX 75266
1-800-222-7542

Sentry Life Insurance Co.
Senior Care Services, Inc.
Suite 205
10700 West Highway 55
Plymouth, MN 55441
1-800-328-4827 ext. 1069

Transport Life Ins. Co.
714 Main Street
Fort Worth, TX 76102
817/390-8000

Union Bankers
2551 Elm Street
Dallas, TX 75221
214/939-0821

Union Fidelity
4850 Street Road
Trevose, PA 19049
1-800-523-5758

Washington Square Life Ins.
1600 Market Street
Philadelphia, PA 19101
1-800-654-7796

World Insurance Co.
P.O. Box 128
Omaha, NE 68102
402/342-1402

World Life & Health Ins. Co.
of PA
215 West Church Road
King of Prussia, PA 19406
1-800-523-1260

Note: The companies listed all meet the National Association of Insurance Commissioners' Model Act definition of a long-term-care policy. The table does not include all companies selling long-term insurance products.

SOURCE: Health Insurance Association of America. Reprinted with permission.

Keep in mind that, though ratings can be helpful, and *Consumer Reports* rankings are most thorough, you should not accept them blindly. A lesser-ranked policy may be best for you or your parent because of particular needs and finances. In addition, since the types of private long-term-care insurance policies are changing rapidly, ratings good one day may be out-of-date the next.

As you collect information about available policies, you will probably get a sense that these policies are helpful to some people but not worth the expense for others. Despite increased promotion and public understanding, Brookings Institution (a nationally known think-tank) predicts that twenty years from now private long-term-care insurance will still cover only a small portion—about 10 percent—of the nation's nursing-home bill. Most older Americans will still need to utilize the planning techniques discussed in this book in order to protect their savings.

Private Insurance Rip-offs

As discussed earlier, many Americans have been tricked into purchasing unnecessary private insurance coverage (whether Medigap or long-term-care coverage) by deceptive advertising and high-pressure sales. Some salespeople have even taken money from elderly citizens and disappeared, without providing any insurance coverage at all.

Here are some tips to protect people from insurance deception:

- Don't buy insurance just because a star like Michael Landon says it's the right thing to do. He's being paid to endorse the product, and his advice to consumers is not necessarily based on experience or conviction.
- Don't assume any insurance policy is sponsored or endorsed by the federal or state government or an established senior advocacy organization. Some policies use deceptive names, and some salespeople even falsely tell consumers that their policy is offered under government auspices. *No* Medigap or long-term-care policy is offered by a state or the federal government, and only a very few group policies are sold by legitimate senior advocacy organizations (like the AARP).
- Stay away from insurance for specific illnesses, such as cancer. These policies are often sold by scare tactics. Their protection is narrow, applying only to certain terrifying diseases, and such policies also tend to duplicate existing coverage under Medicare and standard Medigap policies.
- Don't duplicate coverage. Ten policies offering identical coverage will cost ten times more than one such policy but will not provide ten times more protection.
- Just because a policy does not require a medical exam does *not* mean that it provides coverage for preexisting illnesses. As discussed before, insurers will ask about an applicant's health; if the questions aren't answered fully and honestly, the applicant risks cancellation of a granted policy.
- Don't be misled by glittering generalities about the policy costs, such as "low weekly rates." Figure out the monthly and annual costs and compare policies using the checklist in this chapter.
- If you decide to buy private insurance, the check should be made out to the insurance company, *not* the agent. There have been cases, with checks made out to agents, where people have wound up without check, agent, or coverage.
- Don't rely on oral promises made by a salesperson. If it's not in writing, it's not in the policy.

11 | A Living Will Can Protect

Peace of Mind and Savings

Consider this situation:

Your parent is struck with a catastrophic injury or illness, and the doctors can offer no hope for recovery. The only way to prolong his or her life is with artificial "heroic" measures, perhaps sustaining the parent in a nursing facility. This is a dreaded scenario, but unfortunately one that individuals sometimes must face.

Does your parent want to make his or her own choice about whether to live or die under certain conditions? If so, *now* is the time for your parent to make those wishes known.

By preparing a living will and/or a durable power of attorney, a parent can help ensure that his or her wishes will be followed. Although a living will is not designed primarily to save money, it can protect and relieve a family of the terrible emotional burden and financial devastation of unwanted long-term care.

A living will is a piece of paper that tells one's family, doctors, and friends what medical treatment he or she wants—or doesn't want—if he or she becomes terminally ill or seriously injured and cannot make or communicate decisions regarding treatment.

A living will is *not* the same as a will or a living trust. Don't be confused. A will deals with the distribution of money and property after a person dies; a living trust can be used to hold and manage money and property during a person's lifetime or after his or her death. Both are completely different from a living will, and neither addresses the issue of withholding or terminating medical treatment.

Why Have a Living Will?

Most states have passed living will laws designed to protect a patient's right to refuse medical treatment. In those states, a living will is recognized as a legally enforceable document and can ensure that a doctor who abides by a patient's wishes not to be kept alive on life supports will be insulated from any possible liability.

Even in those few states without living will laws, a living will can still be useful. Without state legislation, judges are often left to determine what an unconscious patient would have wanted if he or she could speak. In making such a decision, a judge is likely to give weight to a living will, even though it is not legally recognized by specific legislation.

If your parent (or you) wants to exercise his or her right to make choices concerning health care in the event of incapacity, and at the same time spare the rest of the family the terrible trauma of making life-and-death decisions, a living will is essential. Your parent should make out a living will *now*, while he or she is still of sound mind and capable of communicating. If your parent later becomes terminally ill, *another* living will should be prepared—that way, nobody will be able to discount the first will's validity by saying that it was executed while your parent was healthy and that his or her feelings may have changed after becoming ill.

After making out a living will, your parent should give copies to his or her family, doctors, clergy, and closest friends, and should carry one in the glove compartment of his or her car. If your parent goes into the hospital, copies should be given to the doctors and nurses and included on the parent's chart. By doing that, your parent will enhance the chance that his or her living will will be considered when actually needed.

If your parent ever decides to cancel a living will, an oral revocation is legally sufficient in most states. Still, to avoid any mixups, all copies of that will previously given out should be returned so they can be destroyed. Your parent should also write out a statement, witnessed by two people, that his or her living will is canceled. This should eliminate any possible confusion over his or her true wishes.

On page 81 is a Living Will Declaration form recommended for use in those states that have *not* adopted living will statutes (those states not included in Table 19). Although not legally binding on the courts, this Living Will Declaration should be helpful in communicating your parent's wishes concerning medical treatment. The form is followed by Instructions/Explanation to clarify the terms of the document, so that your parent understands exactly what it is he or she is signing.

In those states (listed in Table 19) that have living will laws, the Living Will Declaration forms are prescribed by the state. Tables 20 and 21 list witness requirements and other limitations imposed in different states on living wills. Copies of suitable state forms prepared by the Society for the Right to Die are available from the society. For such copies, and for more information about living wills, contact the Society for the Right to Die, 250 West 57th Street, New York, New York 10107, (212) 246-6973.

Can a Durable Power of Attorney Help?

In general, a power of attorney authorizes another person to make decisions and/or act for the maker; many people have used powers of attorney at some time or another. A *durable* power of attorney is the same thing except it continues to be valid even if the maker is incapacitated. Use of durable powers of attorney in connection with management of a person's financial affairs is discussed in Chapter 7.

Some experts suggest that a person could use a durable power of attorney as a legally effective means to give someone else a "proxy" to make decisions about medical treatment on the maker's behalf. Still, many states have not yet decided whether durable powers of attorney may be used in connection with medical treatment and, particularly, with the termination of treatment. At the time of this writing, only seven states—California, Colorado, Idaho, Maine, Pennsylvania, Rhode Island, and Utah—have adopted legislation specifically authorizing use of a durable power of attorney for health care decisions. In New York, the state attorney general issued an opinion in 1984 that cast doubt in that state on the use of durable powers of attorney in connection with health care decisions.

When and if permitted to be applicable to health care decisions, durable powers of attorney can offer more flexibility than living wills. Specifically, they can be used to make decisions for someone who becomes incapable of making his or her own decisions even if not terminally ill.

In conclusion, if an individual wants to express his or her wishes concerning medical intervention and the right to die with dignity, he or she should plan ahead by making a living will and/or a durable power of attorney.

TABLE 19

States with Living Will Laws

Alabama	Mississippi
Alaska	Missouri
Arizona	Montana
Arkansas	Nevada
California	New Hampshire
Colorado	New Mexico
Connecticut	North Carolina
Delaware	Oklahoma
District of Columbia	Oregon
Florida	South Carolina
Georgia	Tennessee
Hawaii	Texas
Idaho	Utah
Illinois	Vermont
Indiana	Virginia
Iowa	Washington
Kansas	West Virginia
Louisiana	Wisconsin
Maine	Wyoming
Maryland	

SOURCE: *You and Your Living Will*, published by the Society for the Right to Die, undated. Reprinted by permission.

TABLE 20

Witness Requirements for Living Will Declarations

STATE	WITNESS MAY NOT BE:				
	Related to Your Parent by Blood or Marriage	Heir or Claimant to Your Parent's Estate	Your Parent's Physician	Employed by Your Parent's Health Care Facility	Responsible for Your Parent's Health Care Costs
Alabama	X	X			X
Alaska	X				
Arizona	X	X			X
California[a]	X	X	X	X	
Colorado		X	or any M.D.	or co-patient	
Delaware[a]	X	X		X	X
District of Columbia[a]	X	X	X	X	X
Florida	(one of two witnesses)				
Georgia[b]	X	X	X	X	X
Hawaii	X or adoption		X	X	
Idaho	X	X	X	X	
Illinois	X	X			X
Indiana	only parents, spouse, and children	X			X
Kansas	X	X			X
Louisiana	X	X	X	or co-patient	
Maryland	X	X	X	X	X
Mississippi	X	X	X		
Nevada	X	X	X	X	
New Hampshire[b]	X	X	X		
North Carolina	X	X	X	X	
Oklahoma	X	X	X	or co-patient	X
Oregon[c]	X	X	X	X	
South Carolina[d]	X	X	X	X	X
Tennessee	X	X	X	X	
Texas	X	X	X	or co-patient	
Utah	X	X	X	X	X
Vermont	X	X		X	
Virginia	X				
Washington	X	X	X	X	
West Virginia	X	X	X	X	X
Wisconsin	X	X	X	X	
Wyoming	X	X			X

[a]Nursing-home patient requires patient advocate or ombudsman as witness.
[b]Nursing-home patient requires medical director as witness.
[c]Nursing-home patient requires an individual designated by Department of Human Resources as witness.
[d]South Carolina requires three witnesses and a notary. For a hospital or nursing-home patient, one witness must be an ombudsman.

SOURCE: Table 4, *A Matter of Choice: Planning Ahead for Health Care Decisions*, a publication of the American Association of Retired Persons, prepared for use by United States Senators John Heinz and John Glenn. Copyright © 1987, American Association of Retired Persons. Reprinted with permission.

LIVING WILL DECLARATION

To My Family, Doctors, and All Those Concerned with My Care:

     I, _____, being of sound mind, make this statement as a directive to be followed if I become unable to participate in decisions regarding my medical care.

     If I should be in an incurable or irreversible mental or physical condition with no reasonable expectation of recovery, I direct my attending physician to withhold or withdraw treatment that merely prolongs my dying. I further direct that treatment be limited to measures to keep me comfortable and to relieve pain.

     These directions express my legal right to refuse treatment. Therefore, I expect my family, doctors, and everyone concerned with my care to regard themselves as legally and morally bound to act in accord with my wishes, and in so doing to be free of any legal liability for having followed my directions.

     I especially do not want: _____

_____

_____

_____

     Other instructions/comments: _____

_____

_____

_____

_____

_____

_____

_____

_____

_____

_____

Proxy Designation Clause: Should I become unable to communicate my instructions as stated above, I designate the following person to act in my behalf:

Name: _____

Address: _____

If the person I have named above is unable to act in my behalf, I authorize the following person to do so:

Name: _____

Address: _____

_____

Signed: _____   Date: _____

Witness: _____   Witness: _____

Living Will Declaration

Instructions/Explanation

The explanations that follow should provide you with a clear understanding of the terms used in the Living Will Declaration.

Introduction: The opening sentence addresses the Living Will Declaration to your family and doctors because they are the ones most likely to be faced with making decisions concerning your medical treatment if you can't make those decisions.

In the first blank, fill in your name and address.

The next two paragraphs are most important, setting forth your directions regarding medical treatment. The first limits the withholding or withdrawal of treatment to situations in which there is *no* reasonable expectation that you will recover. In those situations, you are directing your physician to allow you to die with dignity.

The next paragraph is optional. It provides space for you to list specific treatments you do not want, such as cardiac resuscitation, mechanical respiration, and artificial feeding/fluids by tubes. If you leave this section blank, your general statements in the paragraphs above should still protect your wishes.

The next paragraph allows you to state any other instructions or comments. For example, you may want to add instructions for care you *do* want, such as pain medication, nursing care, and other treatment designed to keep you as comfortable and free of pain as possible. You also might want to

specify here a desire to be allowed to die at home if possible.

Proxy Designation Clause: This is your designation of someone you trust to see that your wishes are carried out. Again, this is optional; it serves as a second protection to ensure that your wishes are fulfilled. If you do designate a proxy, talk to that person first to explain your desires and make sure that person will carry them out.

Finally, sign and date the Living Will Declaration before two adult witnesses, who should also sign. If possible, the witnesses should not be your physicians, relatives, or beneficiaries of your estate. (See Table 20.)

After signing the Living Will Declaration, keep it with your important papers at home. Give copies to doctors, family, and proxies—all those who someday might have to use it. And discuss it with them, so that they know exactly how you feel. Have your physician include a copy in your medical records.

You may also want to keep a card in your wallet stating that you've signed a living will and noting where it is located. Don't keep it in your safe-deposit box, because access is too limited.

Finally, review your living will from time to time. If it continues to express your intent, initial and date it each time. That way, anyone reading it will know that you haven't changed your mind.

TABLE 21

Special Limitations on Living Will Declarations

STATE	CATEGORICALLY MAY NOT WITHHOLD FOOD AND FLUIDS	TERMINAL CONDITION MUST BE MEDICALLY CERTIFIED	TO BE BINDING, MUST BE SIGNED AFTER TERMINAL DIAGNOSIS
Alabama		X	
Alaska		X	
Arizona	X	X	
Arkansas		X	
California[a]		X	X
Colorado		X	
Connecticut		X	
Delaware		X	
District of Columbia		X	
Florida	X	X	
Georgia		X	
Hawaii		X	X
Idaho			
Illinois	X	X	
Indiana	X[b]	X	
Iowa	X	X	
Kansas		X	
Louisiana		X	
Maine	X	X	
Maryland	X	X	
Mississippi		X	
Missouri	X	X	
Montana		X	
New Hampshire	X	X	
New Mexico		X	
North Carolina		X	
Oklahoma		X	X
Oregon	X[c]	X	
South Carolina	X	X	
Tennessee	X	X	
Texas		X	
Utah	X[d]	X	
Virginia		X	
Washington		X	
West Virginia		X	
Wisconsin	X	X	
Wyoming	X	X	

[a]Declaration valid for five years.
[b]May not withhold "appropriate" nourishment and hydration.
[c]May withhold if your parent cannot tolerate.
[d]Unless your parent specifically authorizes.

SOURCE: Adapted from Table 5, *A Matter of Choice: Planning Ahead for Health Care Decisions*, a publication of the American Association of Retired Persons, prepared for use by United States Senators John Heinz and John Glenn, copyright © 1987, American Association of Retired Persons, reprinted with permission; and from *Checklist Chart of Living Will Laws*, Society for the Right to Die, also reprinted with permission.

12 A Lawyer Can Be Helpful
If You Pick the Right One

An elderly woman went to see her lawyer about a will. After she nervously went through the list of gifts she wanted to make, the lawyer said, "Don't worry, just leave it all to me." She immediately responded, "I guess you're right—you'll get it all anyway." For many of us, this joke has more than a ring of truth to it.

No one wants to spend a fortune on legal fees, but a lawyer experienced in Medicaid matters *can* be helpful, particularly if you (or a loved one) would like personalized guidance concerning planning techniques. The right lawyer can offer invaluable assistance and, in the long run, save you money.

How Do You Find the Right Lawyer?

Finding a lawyer is rarely a problem. The challenge is finding the *right* one—ideally an individual who's experienced in Medicaid planning and sensitive to the needs of the elderly. Here are eight tips to consider when shopping for an attorney:

1. Ask your friends; perhaps they've already used a lawyer for estate planning or Medicaid planning advice. If they recommend their personal injury lawyer, that lawyer probably is *not* the right attorney to advise you about Medicaid matters, although he or she might be able to recommend someone who can.
2. Ask other professionals you trust; your doctor, clergyman, or banker might know an experienced Medicaid lawyer. These people often work with such lawyers and may know a good one.
3. If there's a law school nearby, ask for a professor who handles probate or estate planning. Some professors will be happy to recommend a lawyer to you.
4. If you or your parent works for a company that hires outside lawyers, call that lawyer and ask for a referral. Because a member of your family works for one of his clients, he is likely to want to make you happy and may help find an experienced Medicaid lawyer if he doesn't already know one.
5. Local bar associations often offer referral services that can provide names of attorneys. These should be used only as a last resort. Lawyers generally get on such lists by paying a small fee—bar associations rarely do any screening at all—so you have no assurance about the competency or expertise of a lawyer recommended through a referral service.
6. Don't pick a lawyer at random from the telephone book. That's like playing Russian roulette.
7. Don't rely on general advertising. Anyone can advertise—regardless of ability or experience.
8. Be wary of referrals from anyone who will benefit from a referral. For example, a real estate agent, accountant, or financial planner may work with one or two lawyers; they refer business to the lawyer, and the lawyer refers business to them. Sometimes these referrals are fine, because the referror can benefit from your satisfaction; however, your or your parent's needs may not be the primary concern in such a situation.

How Do You Choose a Lawyer?

Once you have a list of names, how do you pick the right one? First try to narrow the field by finding out as much as possible about each lawyer's reputation and experience. Ask lawyers you know if they are familiar with the names recommended to you. You can also check the *Martindale-Hubbell Directory*, available in most libraries.

The *Martindale-Hubbell Directory* lists most lawyers in the country and gives some helpful information about them. Unfortunately, it is not the easiest book to decipher. Here's how to read it:

1. Choose the volume that includes the state in which the lawyer practices.
2. Find the roster of lawyers in the state near the beginning of the volume.
3. Find the city in which the lawyer practices and locate his or her name.
4. Immediately following the attorney's name are his or her date of birth and date of first admission to the bar.
5. Sometimes a rating, indicated by one or two lowercase letters, will be next. An explanation of this rating can be found below.
6. Next is a "C." followed by a number and an "L." followed by a number; respectively, these indicate the lawyer's college and law school. Now turn to the beginning of the volume to find the list showing what school is represented by each number. The first degrees received are also usually included (i.e., B.A., J.D.).
7. Finally, some names are followed by the name of a law firm in brackets. If an "A" precedes the firm's name, that indicates the lawyer is an associate (an employee of the office, not a partner). If a firm's name is listed in brackets, there may be additional information about its attorneys in the biographical section later in the volume.

Here's an example of how the listing works:

Smith, John.......'53 '77 a v C.821 B.A. L.569 J.D. [Hahn L. & P.]

John Smith was born in 1953 and graduated from law school in 1977. "C.821 B.A." means that he earned his Bachelor's Degree at Swarthmore College; "L. 569 J.D." means that he received his law degree at New York University. "[Hahn L. & P.]" is shorthand for Hahn Loeser & Parks, his law firm.

Since there is a law firm listed, you can look to the biographical section of the volume for additional information. For John Smith, you might find:

JOHN D. SMITH, born Cleveland, Ohio, June 2, 1953; admitted to bar, 1977, Maryland; 1979, District of Columbia, Ohio, U.S. District Court for the District of Columbia and U.S. Court of Appeals for the District of Columbia Circuit. Education: Swarthmore College (B.A., cum laude, 1974); New York University (J.D., cum laude, 1977). Order of the Coif. Root-Tilden Scholar. Associate Editor, New York University Law Review, 1976–1977. Law Clerk to Honorable Aubrey E. Robinson, Jr., Chief Judge, U.S. District Court for the District of Columbia. Author: "You and the Law," columns in the Cleveland Plain Dealer, 1982–, Cincinnati Enquirer, 1984– and Columbus Dispatch, 1985–. Member Cleveland (Chairman, Young Lawyers Section, 1983–1984; Member, Board of Trustees, 1983–1984), Ohio State and American (Member, Executive Council, Young Lawyers Division, 1986–1987) Bar Association.

The *Martindale-Hubbell Directory* also rates lawyers, based on their legal ability and ethical standards, by surveying lawyers and judges in the area where the lawyer practices. These are the only nationally recognized lawyer ratings.

The legal ability ratings are "a" (very high), "b" (high), and "c" (fair). These ratings are supposedly based upon the lawyer's ability, experience, nature and length of practice. The ethical rating is a "v" (very high). There is no other ethical rating available; a lawyer receives either a "v" or nothing. So if the lawyer you are considering has an "a v" rating (like John Smith), take that as a major plus. Of course, many lawyers, good and bad, are not rated by the *Martindale-Hubbell Directory*. The absence of a rating doesn't necessarily mean a lawyer is unqualified.

Interviewing and Comparison Shopping

Once you have narrowed the list, you should interview the lawyers remaining. Most lawyers will meet without charging a fee for the initial conference. If a lawyer insists on charging, you should cross him or her off the list.

Upon arriving at a lawyer's office, you should try

not to let the surroundings affect your judgment. A beautiful office might mean that the lawyer got rich from doing great work for clients, but it might also mean that the lawyer's mother is wealthy and decorated the office for him, or that the lawyer made a lot of money by overcharging clients.

Nor should you be misled by fancy-looking certificates on the walls. Some of the worst lawyers have the most impressive wall coverings. For example, the lawyer may prominently display a certificate stating that he or she has been admitted to practice before the local federal court or even the United States Supreme Court. Don't be fooled—any lawyer can get one of those with a minimal fee and a few references from lawyers in town. Diplomas may be a little more helpful, showing what schools the lawyer has attended. A certificate from the Order of the Coif means that the lawyer graduated at the top of his or her law school class.

Following is a questionnaire you can take when interviewing prospective lawyers.

LAWYER INTERVIEW QUESTIONNAIRE

1. How many people have you counseled on Medicaid matters in the past five years?
   Answer: _____

2. How many Medicaid Trusts and/or durable powers of attorney have you prepared in the past five years?
   Answer: _____

3. Will you give me a list of references—clients whom you've counseled on Medicaid matters? (Then call them, just as you would if you were hiring a painter. If the lawyer refuses to provide references, look elsewhere.)
   Answer: _____

4. Are you familiar with the details of the Medicare Catastrophic Coverage law?
   Answer: _____

5. What outside activities do you participate in? (If the lawyer teaches estate/probate law at a law school, that is a positive recommendation. The fact that he might be active in his church is nice but not pertinent to you.)
   Answer: _____

6. With whom do you consult on legal questions you're not sure about? (A lawyer should have other experienced attorneys either in the office or in the community with whom he or she consults when necessary. No lawyer knows everything; if a lawyer tells you otherwise, look elsewhere.)
   Answer: _____

7. Are you the person who will handle my matter, or will you pass it off to someone else? (You may actually be better off if a younger, lower-priced attorney in the office handles the matter, as long as he or she will be well supervised.)
   Answer: _____

8. Will you keep me informed about the progress of my matter (i.e., preparation of trusts, etc.) on a regular basis?
   Answer: _____

9. What will your fee be?
   Answer: _____

10. Will you provide me with regular, detailed billings?
    Answer: _____

How the lawyer answers the questions is as important as *what* is said. You should feel comfortable with the lawyer, confident in his or her abilities, and satisfied that he or she understands your or your parent's needs and will answer your questions clearly and without making you feel stupid or that you are wasting his or her time.

Conclusion

A variety of tools to safeguard family nest eggs, within the existing laws, have been presented in this book. To summarize and exemplify these tools, here are two final series of guidelines that draw upon the full range of this book's various alternatives.

Master Checklist to Protect Assets

The following steps can help an elderly person protect his or her assets from being wiped out by catastrophic long-term-care costs.

OPTIONS AVAILABLE BEFORE ONE REQUIRES LONG-TERM CARE

While you are healthy and not in need of long-term care, you should:

- Prepare a durable power of attorney for a spouse and/or child, giving it to a third person to hold, if possible. This allows you maximum planning flexibility and should *guarantee* that you incur no loss greater than about $60,000 (two and one-half years of nursing-home costs).
- Consider setting up a Medicaid Trust. A Medicaid Trust allows you to preserve your assets *without* transferring them to children or others and ensures that the income from those assets would be available if you were to enter and then return home from a nursing home.
- Check out long-term-care insurance policies.

You may find one that offers important protection at a price that makes sense.
- Consider making a living will.
- Consider making tax-free gifts to children and/or others, to reduce the amount of assets available to a nursing home.
- Consider transferring your home to children and/or others, but retaining a life estate. That guarantees you the right to live there.

OPTIONS AVAILABLE WHEN ONE ENTERS A NURSING HOME AND LEAVES A SPOUSE AT HOME

Should you have to go into a nursing home, leaving a spouse at home:

- You should, where practical, change money into exempt assets, such as a home, household goods, personal effects, car, property producing income for support, life insurance, and burial plots and expenses. Exempt assets, other than the house, may then be transferred to others.
- You should transfer the house into the name of your spouse-at-home, and at the same time the spouse-at-home should change his or her will so that the house won't revert to you (and then to the nursing home) if he or she dies.
- You may transfer assets to your spouse-at-home, who may then transfer those assets to children or others. This gets assets out of the nursing home's reach without running afoul of transfer-eligibility rules.
- Your spouse-at-home may protect both assets

and income by getting a divorce. In some states, a support order can protect income for the spouse-at-home without actually going through a divorce.

OPTIONS AVAILABLE WHEN AN UNMARRIED PERSON ENTERS A NURSING HOME

Should you be an unmarried person entering a nursing home, you should:

- Where practical, consider transferring money into exempt assets, particularly a house. However, in many states, the protection for a house disappears soon after an unmarried person enters a nursing home.
- Consider transferring exempt assets other than the house to children and/or others. These transfers will not violate the transfer-ineligibility rules.
- Consider transferring nonexempt assets directly to children and/or others or you may pay your children for services they have provided. Also consider transferring the house, but only if the protection for it will disappear soon after you enter a nursing home. Although these transfers won't help you qualify for Medicaid for two and one-half years, at least you can minimize losses.

· · · · · · · · · · ·

Sample Medicaid Plans

Following are four sample Medicaid plans illustrating how one's parents may employ the strategies described in this book to protect their life savings.

SITUATION 1

Your parents own a home and have additional assets (CDs and stock) totaling $100,000. Some assets are owned jointly with rights of survivorship, others are owned individually. Your parents' income is about $25,000 annually, an amount sufficient for them to live on even excluding interest and dividends.

They have three children, Joe, who lives in town, and two away. They have a good relationship with all three, but are closest with Joe because of his proximity. Your parents' wills are simple, leaving everything first to each other and then to the children in equal shares.

Now your father has become seriously ill. Although he's mentally competent, he may soon have to enter a nursing home. Here are two possible plans that could benefit your parents in this situation:

PLAN 1

1. Each parent should prepare one durable power of attorney naming the other as attorney-in-fact and a second naming Joe as attorney-in-fact. They could also make durable powers of attorney naming each of their other children, if necessary to maintain family harmony. They should give the durable powers of attorney to a third person (like their lawyer) to hold until it becomes necessary to use them.

2. Your father should consider making a living will.

3. They should transfer the house into your mother's name, and your mother may empty joint accounts and use the money to open accounts in her own name, but they should not transfer assets presently in your father's name alone until your father has entered a nursing home.

4. After entering a nursing home, your father should transfer the remaining assets into your mother's name alone.

5. After the assets have been transferred into your mother's name, she may then choose to make tax-free transfers to the children, since she has enough income to live on exclusive of interest income and dividends from CDs and stock. However, she could be putting herself at risk in the event of an emergency or the death of her husband, unless she is sure her children would care for her if necessary.

6. As an alternative to step 5, your mother may consider placing the assets into a Medicaid Trust, protecting the income yielded by those assets for her (and your father if he recovers enough to return home).

7. After your father enters a nursing home, your

mother should change her will, removing him as beneficiary.

PLAN 1A

1. Each parent should prepare durable powers of attorney as in Plan 1.
2. Your father should consider making a living will.
3. Assume the house has a $50,000 mortgage. That could be paid off by selling some stock or cashing in a CD when it becomes due.
4. Your parents could also buy a new refrigerator and stove to replace the ones they've had for fifteen years.
5. The remaining steps 3–5 of Plan 1 could be followed.

SITUATION 2

Your father passed away many years ago, and your mother has needed full-time care for the last few years. You moved in with her two years ago and have been helping to dress, bathe, and feed her. But you are now sixty-three and won't be able to manage all of your mother's needs for much longer. You are the only living child.

Besides the house, your mother has about $50,000 in several accounts, all of which have your name on them too.

PLAN 2

1. Your mother should prepare a durable power of attorney naming you as attorney-in-fact.
2. Your mother could consider establishing a Medicaid Trust, depending on how long you think you'll be able to maintain her at home. The longer you can maintain her at home, the more likely she'll be able to avoid Medicaid ineligibility under the two-and-a-half-year transfer-ineligibility rule.
3. Your mother could "invest" some or all of her cash in the house, paying off a mortgage, making improvements, and/or purchasing household goods.
4. Your mother could then transfer the house to you. This transfer can be done before she goes into a nursing home and not affect her Medicaid eligibility, because you have lived in the house for two years helping your mother stay out of an institution.

5. Your mother can set aside funds for her funeral expenses and burial plots for her and you.
6. Your mother may invest in other exempt assets (page 18–19), which could be transferred to you.

SITUATION 3

Your parents are both in their fifties and doing quite well. They want to plan ahead to avoid impoverishment by nursing-home costs.

They presently own a home, and their remaining assets total about $150,000. They have three children.

PLAN 3

1. Your parents should make durable powers of attorney for each other and, probably, for at least one of the children.
2. Your parents should look closely at long-term-care insurance policies. At their age, the policies may be available at a reasonable premium.
3. Your parents may consider establishing Medicaid Trusts if they are concerned about jeopardizing their financial stability by making transfers of assets in the future.
4. They may consider making gifts to their children. However, the drawback to this (and, to a lesser extent, with the Medicaid Trust) is that your parents may need to use their assets in the future.
5. They should consider "equalizing" at least some of their assets between themselves.
6. They should consider making living wills.

SITUATION 4

Your father has assets of $150,000 and is living off the income from them. He is currently healthy but is worried about what may happen if he becomes ill. He has three children, but he doesn't want to give away his assets to them while he is alive because he doesn't want to place himself in any financial jeopardy.

PLAN 4

1. Your father should seriously consider setting up a Medicaid Trust, perhaps naming one of

the children as trustee. That way, his income stream would not be jeopardized while he is alive, and his estate would be secured for his children after he died. If he enters a nursing home and subsequently recovers enough to be released, his assets would be preserved and the income from those assets would still be available.

2. He should check out long-term-care insurance policies.

3. He should consider making a living will.

. . . .

No problem facing older Americans and their families today is more severe than that posed by the catastrophic costs of long-term care, and our government has done little to address the roots of the problem.

If we care about the quality of our lives and the lives of our parents and grandparents, we must all continue to pressure our elected officials to act in the best interests of the elderly. We will all be better off once the politicians finally decide to adopt a system that allows older Americans to obtain long-term care without having to impoverish themselves and their families.

Until that time comes, families are on their own and must protect themselves. With the tips provided in this book, older Americans should be able to "avoid the Medicaid trap" and protect their savings from catastrophic care costs.

Appendix A
Durable Power of Attorney Forms

In Chapter 7 I discussed the usage and advantages of a durable power of attorney. The first form that follows was prepared by Barbara Gilder Quint for *Family Circle* magazine (June 1, 1987). She drafted it for use in every state except Florida, Missouri, North Carolina, and Wyoming. If you live in Wyoming, a similar preprinted form is available in stationery stores for about one dollar. Subsequently in this appendix are durable power of attorney forms applicable to the other states. Also included are forms provided by the state legislatures in New York, California, Minnesota, and Connecticut. While the *Family Circle* form was drafted to be acceptable in these four states as well as most others, there are some differences, and third parties who may be asked to rely on the use of a durable power of attorney will probably be more familiar with their own state's version.

Each form is followed by a set of Instructions/Explanation designed to help clarify the form's provisions.

DURABLE GENERAL POWER OF ATTORNEY

STATE OF _____

COUNTY OF _____

        Know all Men by These Presents, which are intended to constitute a DURABLE GEN-ERAL POWER OF ATTORNEY,

That I _____
(Name of principal)

_____
(Address of principal)

do hereby appoint _____
(Name of agent)

_____
(Address of agent)
and

_____
(Name of agent if more than one agent is designated)

_____
(Address of agent if more than one agent is designated)

My Attorney(s)-in-Fact TO ACT (jointly) (severally), as my true and lawful Attorney(s)-in-Fact, for me and in my name, place and stead:

    (A) Power with Respect to Accounts and Instruments. To establish or open accounts, certificates of deposit and any other form of account or instrument for me with financial institutions of any kind; to modify, terminate, make deposits to and write checks on and endorse checks for or make withdrawals from all accounts in my name or with respect to which I am an authorized signatory; to negotiate, endorse or transfer any checks or other instruments with respect to any such accounts; to contract for any services rendered by any financial institution; and to add property to any trust agreement created by me.

    (B) Power with Respect to Safe-Deposit Boxes. To contract with any institution for the maintenance of a safe-deposit box in my name; to have access to all safe-deposit boxes in my name or with respect to which I am an authorized signatory; to add to and remove from the contents of any such safe-deposit box and to terminate any and all contracts for such boxes.

    (C) Power to Sell and Buy. To sell and buy personal, intangible or mixed property, upon such terms and conditions as my Attorney(s)-in-Fact deems appropriate; to use any credit card held in my name to make such purchases and to sign such charge slips as may be necessary to use such credit cards; and to repay from any funds belonging to me any money borrowed and to pay for any purchases made or cash advanced using credit cards issued to me.

    (D) Power to Exercise Rights in Securities. To exercise all rights with respect to securities that I now own, or may hereafter acquire; to establish, utilize and terminate brokerage accounts; and to invest and reinvest any of my assets in stocks, common and/or preferred, bonds (including, without limitation, United States Treasury Bonds or other United States government obligations which may be redeemed at par for the purpose of applying the entire amount of principal and accrued interest thereon to the payment of the Federal estate tax, if any, occasioned by my death), notes, debentures, loans, mortgages, common trust funds, or other securities or property, real or personal, upon such terms and conditions as my Attorney(s)-in-Fact deems appropriate.

(E) Power to Borrow Money (including any Insurance Policy Loans). To borrow money for my account upon such terms and conditions as my Attorney(s)-in-Fact may deem appropriate and to secure such borrowing by the granting of security interests in any property or interest in property which I may now or hereafter own; to borrow money upon any life insurance policies owned by me upon my life for any purpose and to grant a security interest in such policy to secure any such loans; and no insurance company shall be under any obligation whatsoever to determine the need for such loan or the application of the proceeds therefrom.

(F) Power with Respect to Real Property. To purchase real property, to manage, maintain and alter all real property belonging to me, and to lease, sell, mortgage, encumber or otherwise dispose of all interests in real property belonging to me, upon such terms and conditions as my Attorney(s)-in-Fact deems appropriate; to renew leases of the same or to execute, acknowledge and deliver leases therefor; to execute deeds of conveyance either with or without covenants of general warranty; to pay and satisfy all mortgages, encumbrances, taxes and assessments that may be a lien or charge upon any of my real property; and to receive rentals from and the proceeds of sale of any of my real property. For purposes of this Durable General Power of Attorney, real property shall include, without limitation, the real property known as _____.

(G) Power to Demand, Compromise and Receive. To demand, arbitrate, settle, sue for, collect, receive, deposit, expand for my benefit, reinvest or make such other appropriate dispositions of, as my Attorney(s)-in-Fact deems appropriate, all cash rights to payments of cash, property (personal, intangible and/or mixed), rights and/or benefits to which I am now or may in the future become entitled, regardless of the identity of the individual or public or private entity involved (and for purposes of receiving Social Security benefits, my Attorney(s)-in-Fact is herewith appointed my "Representative Payee"); to compound, compromise, settle and adjust all claims and demands whatsoever which I may now owe or be liable for; and to utilize all lawful means and methods for such purposes.

(H) Power with Respect to Taxes. To make, prepare, sign and file for me and on my behalf any and all required tax estimates and returns, federal, state or local, as well as any waivers, affidavits, schedules or other forms required or permitted to be filed in connection therewith, and to protest and appeal any assessments or determinations of tax against me which my Attorney(s)-in-Fact deems to have been made without proper warrant.

(I) Power with Respect to Documents. To sign, acknowledge, record and deliver agreements, affidavits, bills of sale, stock powers, deeds, leases, mortgages, notes, receipts, releases, satisfactions, journal entries, certificates and such other documents which may be necessary or convenient in execution of the powers hereinbefore expressly conferred upon my Attorney(s)-in-Fact; to execute and deliver applications for automobile license plates and certificates of title and to endorse for transfer and to deliver certificates of title; and to execute and deliver applications for insurance (including, without limitation, insurance on my life) and to cancel and select the amounts therefor.

(J) Power to Engage Services. To engage the services of and compensate attorneys-at-law, appraisers, accountants, brokers, real estate managers, investment counsel and such other persons as may be proper or convenient to advise and assist in the management, maintenance and disposition of my property.

(K) Power to Incur Obligations. To incur obligations for the maintenance, support, health, care, well-being, comfort and welfare of me and my family and to satisfy such obligations out of my money or property; and to consent on my behalf to medical and surgical procedures.

I further give and grant to my said Attorney(s)-in-Fact full power and authority to do and perform every act necessary to be done in the exercise of any of the foregoing powers as fully as I might or could do if personally present, with full power of substitution and revocation, hereby ratifying and confirming all that my said Attorney(s)-in-Fact shall lawfully do, or cause to be done by virtue hereof.

This instrument may not be changed orally.

This power of attorney is durable and shall not be affected by the subsequent disability or incompetence of the principal or by any lapse of time.

TO INDUCE ANY THIRD PARTY TO ACT HEREUNDER, I HEREBY AGREE THAT ANY THIRD PARTY RECEIVING A DULY EXECUTED COPY OR FACSIMILE OF THIS INSTRUMENT MAY ACT HEREUNDER, AND THAT REVOCATION OR TERMINATION HEREOF SHALL BE INEFFECTIVE AS TO SUCH THIRD PARTY UNLESS AND UNTIL ACTUAL NOTICE OR KNOWLEDGE OF SUCH REVOCATION OF TERMINATION SHALL HAVE BEEN RECEIVED BY SUCH THIRD PARTY AND I FOR MYSELF AND FOR MY HEIRS, EXECUTORS, LEGAL REPRESENTATIVES AND ASSIGNS, HEREBY AGREE TO INDEMNIFY AND HOLD HARMLESS ANY SUCH THIRD PARTY FROM AND AGAINST ANY AND ALL CLAIMS THAT MAY ARISE AGAINST SUCH THIRD PARTY BY REASON OF SUCH THIRD PARTY HAVING RELIED ON THE PROVISIONS OF THIS INSTRUMENT.

In witness whereof, I have hereunto signed my name this _____ day of _____, 19___.

_____
(Signature of Principal)

Specimen Signature of Attorney(s)-in-Fact:

_____

_____

Signed in the presence of:

_____
Witness

_____
Witness

CERTIFICATE OF NOTARY

STATE OF _____)
) SS:
COUNTY OF _____)

On the _____ day of _____, 19___, before me personally came _____, whose identity is well known to me and known to me to be the individual described in and who executed the foregoing instrument, and (he)(she) acknowledged to me that (he)(she) executed the same.

_____
Notary Public

My commission expires:

_____

Durable General Power of Attorney

Instructions/Explanation

As you can see, the Durable General Power of Attorney is filled with legalese. Don't be scared off by this confusing language. The explanations that follow should provide you with a clear understanding of the terms used.

Introduction: At the top left, you will see the words "State of" and "County of." Fill in the name of your state and county. Use a pen, not a pencil.

Below that, fill in your name and address (you are the "principal"—the person making the Durable General Power of Attorney).

On the next lines, fill in the name(s) and address(es) of the person(s) to whom you are giving the Durable General Power of Attorney (called the "Agent(s)" or "Attorney(s)-in-Fact"). Check Table 16 for any special variations in your state. For example, in Florida only certain family members may be appointed as your Attorney(s)-in-Fact.

If you have decided to name more than one Attorney-in-Fact, you must decide whether to strike the word "jointly" or "severally." If you want to require your Attorneys-in-Fact to act together to use the Power of Attorney, you should leave the word "jointly" and strike the word "severally." But if you prefer to allow either of your Attorneys-in-Fact on his/her own to exercise the powers provided in the Power of Attorney, you should strike out the word "jointly" and leave the word "severally."

The following lettered clauses specify broad powers providing your Attorney(s)-in-Fact with latitude to manage your financial affairs. Powers are separately enumerated to avoid any questions about whether you intended to authorize your Attorney(s)-in-Fact to undertake specific actions on your behalf.

Clause A: This clause authorizes your Attorney(s)-in-Fact to open and manage accounts, CDs, and other instruments for you in financial institutions. It also says that your Attorney(s)-in-Fact may add to any trust agreement you may have created.

Clause B: This clause allows your Attorney(s)-in-Fact to maintain and gain access to safe-deposit boxes in your name.

Clause C: This clause permits your Attorney(s)-in-Fact to buy and sell items and to use your credit cards.

Clause D: This clause lets your Attorney(s)-in-Fact invest in securities on your behalf and manage and handle those securities. This is broad enough to allow your Attorney(s)-in-Fact even to vote at stockholders meetings.

Clause E: This clause authorizes your Attorney(s)-in-Fact to borrow money in your name.

Clause F: This clause gives your Attorney(s)-in-Fact broad authority to manage, sell, buy, mortgage, and/or lease real estate, including your home. In the blank, fill in the address(es) of your residence and any other real estate you own. You don't have to change the Durable General Power of Attorney each time you buy or sell real estate. Note that, in the District of Columbia, no deed of conveyance may be executed by an Attorney-in-Fact. Recording requirements vary greatly from state to state.

Clause G: This clause authorizes your Attorney(s)-in-Fact to take any necessary action with respect to rights you have or may have in the future to money or property. It also lets your Attorney(s)-in-Fact handle claims made against you. The term "representative payee" is defined in Chapter 7.

Clause H: This clause gives your Attorney(s)-in-Fact the power to deal with your taxes. Although you might prefer to forget about this, it's important that tax forms be prepared and taxes paid, to avoid possible penalties.

Clause I: This clause spells out the right of your Attorney(s)-in-Fact to sign and execute all sorts of documents on your behalf. It allows your Attorney(s)-in-Fact to handle your applications for license plates, certificates of title, and insurance, too.

Clause J: This clause allows your Attorney(s)-in-Fact to hire specialists to assist in handling your financial affairs.

Clause K: This clause generally authorizes your Attorney(s)-in-Fact to incur and pay bills for your maintenance, support, and care. It also empowers your Attorney(s)-in-Fact to make certain health care decisions.

Closing Paragraphs: The first paragraph following the lettered clauses is a general, catch-all sentence authorizing your Attorney(s)-in-Fact to do anything you could do.

The next line is self-explanatory—you can't change the terms of the document orally.

The final sentence before the paragraph in all capital letters is *crucial* to making your power of attorney *durable,* so that it remains valid at the time you will need it most—during your incapacity.

Some banks and insurance companies have traditionally been unwilling to accept or act on any preprinted power of attorney form that they did not prepare themselves. The last full paragraph printed in all capital letters attempts to deal with this problem. That paragraph will protect third parties relying on the Durable General Power of Attorney and, it is hoped, encourage them to accept this form. However, since there can be no assurance that this will work, you should contact your bank and insurance company to discuss their forms and procedures.

Finally, sign and date the document at the end before two witnesses and a notary. While not every state requires two witnesses and a notary, you won't lose anything by having all three. Have the Attorney(s)-in-Fact sign his or her name under yours. The notary fills in and signs the bottom portion. A notary is authorized by the state or federal government to administer oaths and attest to the authenticity of signatures.

DURABLE FAMILY POWER OF ATTORNEY

STATE OF FLORIDA

COUNTY OF _____

      Know all Men by These Presents, which are intended to constitute a DURABLE FAMILY POWER OF ATTORNEY,

That I _____

                      (Name of principal)

_____

                      (Address of principal)

do hereby appoint _____

                      (Name of agent)

_____

      (Address of agent)

and

_____

(Name of agent if more than one agent is designated)

_____

(Address of agent if more than one agent is designated)

My Attorney(s)-in-Fact TO ACT (jointly) (severally), as my true and lawful Attorney(s)-in-Fact, for me and in my name, place and stead:

      (A) Power with Respect to Accounts and Instruments. To establish or open accounts, certificates of deposit and any other form of account or instrument for me with financial institutions of any kind; to modify, terminate, make deposits to and write checks on and endorse checks for or make withdrawals from all accounts in my name or with respect to which I am an authorized signatory; to negotiate, endorse or transfer any checks or other instruments with respect to any such accounts; to contract for any services rendered by any financial institution; and to add property to any trust agreement created by me.

      (B) Power with Respect to Safe-Deposit Boxes. To contract with any institution for the maintenance of a safe-deposit box in my name; to have access to all safe-deposit boxes in my name or with respect to which I am an authorized signatory; to add to and remove from the contents of any such safe-deposit box and to terminate any and all contracts for such boxes.

      (C) Power to Sell and Buy. To sell and buy personal, intangible or mixed property, upon such terms and conditions as my Attorney(s)-in-Fact deems appropriate; to use any credit card held in my name to make such purchases and to sign such charge slips as may be necessary to use such credit cards; and to repay from any funds belonging to me any money borrowed and to pay for any purchases made or cash advanced using credit cards issued to me.

      (D) Power to Exercise Rights in Securities. To exercise all rights with respect to securities that I now own, or may hereafter acquire; to establish, utilize and terminate brokerage accounts; and to invest and reinvest any of my assets in stocks, common and/or preferred, bonds (including, without limitation, United States Treasury Bonds or other United States government obligations which may be redeemed at par for the purpose of applying the entire amount of principal and accrued interest thereon to the payment of the Federal estate tax, if any, occasioned by my death), notes, debentures, loans, mortgages, common trust funds, or other securities or property, real or personal, upon such terms and conditions as my Attorney(s)-in-Fact deems appropriate.

(E) Power to Borrow Money (including any Insurance Policy Loans). To borrow money for my account upon such terms and conditions as my Attorney(s)-in-Fact may deem appropriate and to secure such borrowing by the granting of security interests in any property or interest in property which I may now or hereafter own; to borrow money upon any life insurance policies owned by me upon my life for any purpose and to grant a security interest in such policy to secure any such loans; and no insurance company shall be under any obligation whatsoever to determine the need for such loan or the application of the proceeds therefrom.

(F) Power with Respect to Real Property. To purchase real property, to manage, maintain and alter all real property belonging to me, and to lease, sell, mortgage, encumber or otherwise dispose of all interests in real property belonging to me, upon such terms and conditions as my Attorney(s)-in-Fact deems appropriate; to renew leases of the same or to execute, acknowledge and deliver leases therefor; to execute deeds of conveyance either with or without covenants of general warranty; to pay and satisfy all mortgages, encumbrances, taxes and assessments that may be a lien or charge upon any of my real property; and to receive rentals from and the proceeds of sale of any of my real property. For purposes of this Durable Family Power of Attorney, real property shall include, without limitation, the real property known as _____.

(G) Power to Demand, Compromise and Receive. To demand, arbitrate, settle, sue for, collect, receive, deposit, expand for my benefit, reinvest or make such other appropriate dispositions of, as my Attorney(s)-in-Fact deems appropriate, all cash rights to payments of cash, property (personal, intangible and/or mixed), rights and/or benefits to which I am now or may in the future become entitled, regardless of the identity of the individual or public or private entity involved (and for purposes of receiving Social Security benefits, my Attorney(s)-in-Fact is herewith appointed my "Representative Payee"); to compound, compromise, settle and adjust all claims and demands whatsoever which I may now owe or be liable for; and to utilize all lawful means and methods for such purposes.

(H) Power with Respect to Taxes. To make, prepare, sign and file for me and on my behalf any and all required tax estimates and returns, federal, state or local, as well as any waivers, affidavits, schedules or other forms required or permitted to be filed in connection therewith, and to protest and appeal any assessments or determinations of tax against me which my Attorney(s)-in-Fact deems to have been made without proper warrant.

(I) Power with Respect to Documents. To sign, acknowledge, record and deliver agreements, affidavits, bills of sale, stock powers, deeds, leases, mortgages, notes, receipts, releases, satisfactions, journal entries, certificates and such other documents which may be necessary or convenient in execution of the powers hereinbefore expressly conferred upon my Attorney(s)-in-Fact; to execute and deliver applications for automobile license plates and certificates of title and to endorse for transfer and to deliver certificates of title; and to execute and deliver applications for insurance (including, without limitation, insurance on my life) and to cancel and select the amounts therefor.

(J) Power to Engage Services. To engage the services of and compensate attorneys-at-law, appraisers, accountants, brokers, real estate managers, investment counsel and such other persons as may be proper or convenient to advise and assist in the management, maintenance and disposition of my property.

(K) Power to Incur Obligations. To incur obligations for the maintenance, support, health, care, well-being, comfort and welfare of me and my family and to satisfy such obligations out of my money or property; and to consent on my behalf to medical and surgical procedures.

I further give and grant to my said Attorney(s)-in-Fact full power and authority to do and perform every act necessary to be done in the exercise of any of the foregoing powers as fully as I might or could do if personally present, with full power of substitution and revocation, hereby ratifying and confirming all that my said Attorney(s)-in-Fact shall lawfully do, or cause to be done by virtue hereof.

Said Attorney(s)-in-Fact is my _____.

Anyone dealing with my Attorney(s)-in-Fact under this Durable Family Power of Attorney may rely on any signed copy, photocopy or similar copy of a signed copy as though it were the original.

This Durable Family Power of Attorney shall not be affected by my future disability, if any, or lapse of time, except as provided by statute. The power conferred on said Attorney(s)-in-Fact by this instrument shall be exercisable from the date specified in this instrument, notwithstanding a later disability or incapacity on my part, unless otherwise provided by statutes of the State of Florida.

All acts done by said Attorney(s)-in-Fact pursuant to the power conferred during any period of my disability or incompetence shall have the same effect and inure to the benefit of and bind me or my heirs, devisees, and personal representatives, as if I were competent and not disabled.

This Durable Family Power of Attorney shall be nondelegable and shall be valid until such time as I shall die, revoke this power, or be adjudged incompetent.

This Durable Family Power of Attorney shall commence on the date of execution hereof.

In witness whereof, I have hereunto signed my name this _____ day of _____, 19____.

_____
(Signature of Principal)

Specimen Signature of Attorney(s)-in-Fact:

_____

Signed in the presence of:

_____

_____
Witness

_____
Witness

CERTIFICATE OF NOTARY

STATE OF _____)
) SS:
COUNTY OF _____)

On the _____ day of _____, 19___, before me personally came

_____, whose identity is well known to me and known to me to be the individual described in and who executed the foregoing instrument, and (he)(she) acknowledged to me that (he)(she) executed the same.

_____
Notary Public

My commission expires:

_____

3

Durable Family Power of Attorney
(Florida)

Instructions/Explanation

As you can readily see, the Durable Family Power of Attorney, adapted for use in Florida, is filled with legalese. Don't be scared off by this confusing language. The explanations that follow should provide you with a clear understanding of the terms used.

Introduction: At the top left, you will see the words "State of Florida" and "County of _____." Fill in the name of your county. Use a pen, not a pencil.

Below that, fill in your name and address (you are the "principal"—the person making the Durable Family Power of Attorney).

On the next lines, fill in the name(s) and address(es) of the person(s) to whom you are giving the Durable Family Power of Attorney (called the "Agent(s)" or "Attorney(s)-in-Fact"). In Florida, your Attorney(s)-in-Fact must be your spouse, parent, adult child, sibling, niece or nephew.

If you have decided to name more than one Attorney-in-Fact, you must decide whether to strike the word "jointly" or "severally." If you want to require your Attorneys-in-Fact to act together to use the Power of Attorney, you should leave the word "jointly" and strike the word "severally." But if you prefer to allow either of your Attorneys-in-Fact on his/her own to exercise the powers provided in the Power of Attorney, you should strike out the word "jointly" and leave the word "severally."

The following lettered clauses specify broad powers providing your Attorney(s)-in-Fact with latitude to manage your financial affairs. Powers are separately enumerated to avoid any questions about whether you intended to authorize your Attorney(s)-in-Fact to undertake specific actions on your behalf.

Clause A: This clause authorizes your Attorney(s)-in-Fact to open and manage accounts, CDs, and other instruments for you in financial institutions. It also says that your Attorney(s)-in-Fact may add to any trust agreement you may have created.

Clause B: This clause allows your Attorney(s)-in-Fact to maintain and gain access to safe-deposit boxes in your name.

Clause C: This clause permits your Attorney(s)-in-Fact to buy and sell items and to use your credit cards.

Clause D: This clause lets your Attorney(s)-in-Fact invest in securities on your behalf and to manage and handle those securities. This is broad enough to allow your Attorney(s)-in-Fact even to vote at stockholders meetings.

Clause E: This clause authorizes your Attorney(s)-in-Fact to borrow money in your name.

Clause F: This clause gives your Attorney(s)-in-Fact broad authority to manage, sell, buy, mortgage, and/or lease real estate, including your home. In the blank, fill in the address(es) of your residence and any other real estate you own. You don't have to change the Durable Family Power of Attorney each time you buy or sell real estate. Recording requirements vary greatly from state to state.

Clause G: This clause authorizes your Attorney(s)-in-Fact to take any necessary action with respect to rights you have or may have in the future to money or property. It also lets your Attorney(s)-in-Fact handle claims made against you. The term "representative payee" is defined in Chapter 7.

Clause H: This clause gives your Attorney(s)-in-Fact the power to deal with your taxes. Although you might prefer to forget about this, it's important that tax forms be prepared and taxes paid, to avoid possible penalties.

Clause I: This clause spells out the right of your Attorney(s)-in-Fact to sign and execute all sorts of documents on your behalf. It allows your Attorney(s)-in-Fact to handle your applications for license plates, certificates of title, and insurance, too.

Clause J: This clause allows your Attorney(s)-in-Fact to hire specialists to assist in handling your financial affairs.

Clause K: This clause generally authorizes your Attorney(s)-in-Fact to incur and pay bills for your maintenance, support, and care. It also empowers your Attorney(s)-in-Fact to make certain health care decisions.

Closing Paragraphs: The first paragraph following the lettered clauses is a general, catch-all sentence authorizing your Attorney(s)-in-Fact to do anything you could do.

The next line contains a blank. Fill in the relationship(s) of your Attorney(s)-in-Fact to you. Remember, your Attorney(s)-in-Fact must be your spouse, parent, adult child, sibling, niece, or nephew.

The next paragraph allows a copy of your signed Durable Family Power of Attorney to be used in place of the original.

The following two paragraphs are *crucial* to making your power of attorney *durable,* so that it remains valid at the time you will need it most—during your incapacity.

The next sentence recognizes that the Durable Family Power of Attorney will be valid until you die, revoke it, or are determined to be incompetent by a judge in a court proceeding. Your Attorney(s)-in-Fact cannot delegate the authority provided under the Durable Family Power of Attorney to others.

The last sentence says that the Durable Family Power of Attorney begins working the moment you sign it.

Finally, sign and date the document at the end before two witnesses and a notary. Have the Attorney(s)-in-Fact sign under your name. The notary fills in and signs the bottom portion. A notary is authorized by the state or federal government to administer oaths and attest to the authenticity of signatures.

DURABLE GENERAL POWER OF ATTORNEY

STATE OF MISSOURI

COUNTY OF _____

        Know all Men by These Presents, which are intended to constitute a DURABLE GENERAL POWER OF ATTORNEY,

That I _____
(Name of principal)

_____
(Address of principal)

do hereby appoint _____
(Name of agent)

_____

(Address of agent)
                   and

_____

(Name of agent if more than one agent is designated)

_____

(Address of agent if more than one agent is designated)

My Attorney(s)-in-Fact TO ACT (jointly) (severally), as my true and lawful Attorney(s)-in-Fact, for me and in my name, place and stead:

    (A) Power with Respect to Accounts and Instruments. To establish or open accounts, certificates of deposit and any other form of account or instrument for me with financial institutions of any kind; to modify, terminate, make deposits to and write checks on and endorse checks for or make withdrawals from all accounts in my name or with respect to which I am an authorized signatory; to negotiate, endorse or transfer any checks or other instruments with respect to any such accounts; to contract for any services rendered by any financial institution; and to add property to any trust agreement created by me.

    (B) Power with Respect to Safe-Deposit Boxes. To contract with any institution for the maintenance of a safe-deposit box in my name; to have access to all safe-deposit boxes in my name or with respect to which I am an authorized signatory; to add to and remove from the contents of any such safe-deposit box and to terminate any and all contracts for such boxes.

    (C) Power to Sell and Buy. To sell and buy personal, intangible or mixed property, upon such terms and conditions as my Attorney(s)-in-Fact deems appropriate; to use any credit card held in my name to make such purchases and to sign such charge slips as may be necessary to use such credit cards; and to repay from any funds belonging to me any money borrowed and to pay for any purchases made or cash advanced using credit cards issued to me.

    (D) Power to Exercise Rights in Securities. To exercise all rights with respect to securities that I now own, or may hereafter acquire; to establish, utilize and terminate brokerage accounts; and to invest and reinvest any of my assets in stocks, common and/or preferred, bonds (including, without limitation, United States Treasury Bonds or other United States government obligations which may be redeemed at par for the purpose of applying the entire amount of principal and accrued interest thereon to the payment of the Federal estate tax, if any, occasioned by my death), notes, debentures, loans, mortgages, common trust funds, or other securities or property, real or personal, upon such terms and conditions as my Attorney(s)-in-Fact deems appropriate.

(E) Power to Borrow Money (including any Insurance Policy Loans). To borrow money for my account upon such terms and conditions as my Attorney(s)-in-Fact may deem appropriate and to secure such borrowing by the granting of security interests in any property or interest in property which I may now or hereafter own; to borrow money upon any life insurance policies owned by me upon my life for any purpose and to grant a security interest in such policy to secure any such loans; and no insurance company shall be under any obligation whatsoever to determine the need for such loan or the application of the proceeds therefrom.

(F) Power with Respect to Real Property. To purchase real property, to manage, maintain and alter all real property belonging to me, and to lease, sell, mortgage, encumber or otherwise dispose of all interests in real property belonging to me, upon such terms and conditions as my Attorney(s)-in-Fact deems appropriate; to renew leases of the same or to execute, acknowledge and deliver leases therefor; to execute deeds of conveyance either with or without covenants of general warranty; to pay and satisfy all mortgages, encumbrances, taxes and assessments that may be a lien or charge upon any of my real property; and to receive rentals from and the proceeds of sale of any of my real property. For purposes of this Durable General Power of Attorney, real property shall include, without limitation,

the real property known as _____.

(G) Power to Demand, Compromise and Receive. To demand, arbitrate, settle, sue for, collect, receive, deposit, expand for my benefit, reinvest or make such other appropriate dispositions of, as my Attorney(s)-in-Fact deems appropriate, all cash rights to payments of cash, property (personal, intangible and/or mixed), rights and/or benefits to which I am now or may in the future become entitled, regardless of the identity of the individual or public or private entity involved (and for purposes of receiving Social Security benefits, my Attorney(s)-in-Fact is herewith appointed my "Representative Payee"); to compound, compromise, settle and adjust all claims and demands whatsoever which I may now owe or be liable for; and to utilize all lawful means and methods for such purposes.

(H) Power with Respect to Taxes. To make, prepare, sign and file for me and on my behalf any and all required tax estimates and returns, federal, state or local, as well as any waivers, affidavits, schedules or other forms required or permitted to be filed in connection therewith, and to protest and appeal any assessments or determinations of tax against me which my Attorney(s)-in-Fact deems to have been made without proper warrant.

(I) Power with Respect to Documents. To sign, acknowledge, record and deliver agreements, affidavits, bills of sale, stock powers, deeds, leases, mortgages, notes, receipts, releases, satisfactions, journal entries, certificates and such other documents which may be necessary or convenient in execution of the powers hereinbefore expressly conferred upon my Attorney(s)-in-Fact; to execute and deliver applications for automobile license plates and certificates of title and to endorse for transfer and to deliver certificates of title; and to execute and deliver applications for insurance (including, without limitation, insurance on my life) and to cancel and select the amounts therefor.

(J) Power to Engage Services. To engage the services of and compensate attorneys-at-law, appraisers, accountants, brokers, real estate managers, investment counsel and such other persons as may be proper or convenient to advise and assist in the management, maintenance and disposition of my property.

(K) Power to Incur Obligations. To incur obligations for the maintenance, support, health, care, well-being, comfort and welfare of me and my family and to satisfy such obligations out of my money or property; and to consent on my behalf to medical and surgical procedures, and to take other actions pertaining to my health.

I further give and grant to my said Attorney(s)-in-Fact full power and authority to do and perform every act necessary to be done in the exercise of any of the foregoing powers as fully as I might or could do if personally present, with full power of substitution and revocation, hereby ratifying and confirming all that my said Attorney(s)-in-Fact shall lawfully do, or cause to be done by virtue hereof.

This instrument may not be changed orally.

This power of attorney is durable as provided for in 486.550 R.S. Mo. et seq. and shall not be affected by the subsequent disability or incompetence of the principal or by any lapse of time; it shall remain in full force and effect until revoked by me.

TO INDUCE ANY THIRD PARTY TO ACT HEREUNDER, I HEREBY AGREE THAT ANY THIRD PARTY RECEIVING A DULY EXECUTED COPY OR FACSIMILE OF THIS INSTRUMENT MAY ACT HEREUNDER, AND THAT REVOCATION OR TERMINATION HEREOF SHALL BE INEFFECTIVE AS TO SUCH THIRD PARTY UNLESS AND UNTIL ACTUAL NOTICE OR KNOWLEDGE OF SUCH REVOCATION OR TERMINATION SHALL HAVE BEEN RECEIVED BY SUCH THIRD PARTY AND I FOR MYSELF AND FOR MY HEIRS, EXECUTORS, LEGAL REPRESENTATIVES AND ASSIGNS, HEREBY AGREE TO INDEMNIFY AND HOLD HARMLESS ANY SUCH THIRD PARTY FROM AND AGAINST ANY AND ALL CLAIMS THAT MAY ARISE AGAINST SUCH THIRD PARTY BY REASON OF SUCH THIRD PARTY HAVING RELIED ON THE PROVISIONS OF THIS INSTRUMENT.

In witness whereof, I have hereunto signed my hand and seal this _____ day of _____, 19___.

_____
(Signature of Principal)

Specimen Signature of Attorney(s)-in-Fact:

_____

Signed in the presence of:

_____

_____
Witness

_____
Witness

CERTIFICATE OF NOTARY

STATE OF _____)
) SS:
COUNTY OF _____)

On the _____ day of _____, 19___, before me personally came _____, whose identity is well known to me and known to me to be the individual described in and who executed the foregoing instrument, and (he)(she) acknowledged to me that (he)(she) executed the same.

_____
Notary Public

My commission expires:

_____

Durable General Power of Attorney
(Missouri)

Instructions/Explanation

The explanations that follow should provide you with a clear understanding of the terms used in the Durable General Power of Attorney.

Introduction: At the top left, you will see the words "State of Missouri" and "County of _____." Fill in the name of your county. Use a pen, not a pencil.

Below that, fill in your name and address (you are the "principal"—the person making the Durable General Power of Attorney).

On the next lines, fill in the name(s) and address(es) of the person(s) to whom you are giving the Durable General Power of Attorney (called the "Agent(s)" or "Attorney(s)-in-Fact").

If you have decided to name more than one Attorney-in-Fact, you must decide whether to strike the word "jointly" or "severally." If you want to require your Attorneys-in-Fact to act together to use the Power of Attorney, you should leave the word "jointly" and strike the word "severally." But if you prefer to allow either of your Attorneys-in-Fact on his/her own to exercise the powers provided in the Power of Attorney, you should strike out the word "jointly" and leave the word "severally."

The following lettered clauses specify broad powers providing your Attorney(s)-in-Fact with latitude to manage your financial affairs. Powers are separately enumerated to avoid any questions about whether you intended to authorize your Attorney(s)-in-Fact to undertake specific actions on your behalf.

Clause A: This clause authorizes your Attorney(s)-in-Fact to open and manage accounts, CDs, and other instruments for you in financial institutions. It also says that your Attorney(s)-in-Fact may add to any trust agreement you may have created.

Clause B: This clause allows your Attorney(s)-in-Fact to maintain and gain access to safe-deposit boxes in your name.

Clause C: This clause permits your Attorney(s)-in-Fact to buy and sell items and to use your credit cards.

Clause D: This clause lets your Attorney(s)-in-Fact invest in securities on your behalf and to manage and handle those securities. This is broad enough to allow your Attorney(s)-in-Fact even to vote at stockholders meetings.

Clause E: This clause authorizes your Attorney(s)-in-Fact to borrow money in your name.

Clause F: This clause gives your Attorney(s)-in-Fact broad authority to manage, sell, buy, mortgage, and/or lease real estate, including your home. In the blank, fill in the address(es) of your residence and any other real estate you own. You don't have to change the Durable General Power of Attorney each time you buy or sell real estate. Recording requirements vary greatly from state to state.

Clause G: This clause authorizes your Attorney(s)-in-Fact to take any necessary action with respect to rights you have or may have in the future to money or property. It also lets your Attorney(s)-in-Fact handle claims made against you. The term "representative payee" is defined in Chapter 7.

Clause H: This clause gives your Attorney(s)-in-Fact the power to deal with your taxes. Although you might prefer to forget about this, it's important that tax forms be prepared and taxes paid, to avoid possible penalties.

Clause I: This clause spells out the right of your Attorney(s)-in-Fact to sign and execute all sorts of documents on your behalf. It allows your Attorney(s)-in-Fact to handle your applications for license plates, certificates of title, and insurance, too.

Clause J: This clause allows your Attorney(s)-in-Fact to hire specialists to assist in handling your financial affairs.

Clause K: This clause generally authorizes your Attorney(s)-in-Fact to incur and pay bills for your maintenance, support, and care. It also empowers your Attorney(s)-in-Fact to make certain health care decisions.

Closing Paragraphs: The first paragraph following the lettered clauses is a general, catch-all sentence authorizing your Attorney(s)-in-Fact to do anything you could do.

The next line is self-explanatory—you can't change the terms of the document orally.

The following sentence is *crucial* to making your power of attorney *durable*, so that it remains valid at the time you will need it most—during your incapacity.

Some banks and insurance companies have traditionally been unwilling to accept or act on any preprinted power of attorney form that they did not prepare themselves. The last full paragraph printed in all capital letters attempts to deal with this problem. That paragraph will protect third parties relying on the Durable General Power of Attorney and, it is hoped, encourage them to accept this form. However, since there can be no assurance that this will work, you should contact your bank and insurance company to discuss their forms and procedures.

Finally, sign and date the document at the end before two witnesses and a notary. Have the Attorney(s)-in-Fact sign his or her name under yours. The notary fills in and signs the bottom portion. A notary is authorized by the state or federal government to administer oaths and attest to the authenticity of signatures.

DURABLE GENERAL POWER OF ATTORNEY

NOTICE: THE POWERS GRANTED BY THIS DOCUMENT ARE BROAD AND SWEEPING. THEY ARE DEFINED IN CHAPTER 32A OF THE NORTH CAROLINA GENERAL STATUTES WHICH EXPRESSLY PERMITS THE USE OF ANY OTHER OR DIFFERENT FORM OF POWER OF ATTORNEY DESIRED BY THE PARTIES CONCERNED.

State Of North Carolina

County Of _____

I, _____, the undersigned, hereby appoint _____ my attorney-in-fact for me and give such person full power to act in my name, place and stead in any way which I myself could do if I were personally present with respect to the following matters as each of them is defined in Chapter 32A of the North Carolina General Statutes to the extent that I am permitted by law to act through an agent. (DIRECTIONS: Initial the line opposite any one or more of the subdivisions as to which the principal desires to give the attorney-in-fact authority.)

(1)   Real property transactions: _____

(2)   Personal property transactions: _____

(3)   Bond, share and commodity transactions: _____

(4)   Banking transactions: _____

(5)   Safe deposits: _____

(6)   Business operating transactions: _____

(7)   Insurance transactions: _____

(8)   Estate transactions: _____

(9)   Personal relationships and affairs: _____

(10) Social security and unemployment: _____

(11) Benefits from military service: _____

(12) Tax: _____

(13) Employment of agents: _____

I also give to such person full power to appoint another to act as my attorney-in-fact and full power to revoke such appointment.

This power of attorney shall not be affected by my subsequent incapacity or mental incompetence.

Dated _____, 19___

_____ (Seal)
Signature

1

STATE OF _____ COUNTY OF _____

     On this ____ day of _____, 19___, personally appeared before me the said named _____ to me known and known to me to be the person described in and who executed the foregoing instrument and he (or she) acknowledged that he (or she) executed the same and being duly sworn by me, made oath that the statements in the foregoing instrument are true.

     My Commission Expires _____

_____

(Signature of Notary Public)
Notary Public (Official Seal)

Durable General Power of Attorney
(North Carolina)

Instructions/Explanation

The explanations that follow should provide you with a clear understanding of the terms used in the Durable General Power of Attorney.

Introduction: At the top left, you will see the words "State Of North Carolina" and "County Of _____." Fill in the name of your county. Use a pen, not a pencil.

Below that, fill in your name and address in the first blank. (You are called the "principal"). In the second blank, fill in the name(s) and address(es) of the person(s) to whom you are giving the Durable General Power of Attorney (called the "Attorney(s)-in-Fact").

Chapter 32A of the North Carolina General Statutes, referred to in your Durable General Power of Attorney, contains the laws governing powers of attorney in North Carolina.

The following numbered lines provide broad powers for your Attorney(s)-in-Fact to manage your affairs. As the directions in the Durable General Power of Attorney indicate, you must initial the lines opposite each power you intend to give to your Attorney(s)-in-Fact. Since you usually can't anticipate every eventuality that might arise, you probably should give your Attorney(s)-in-Fact the widest possible latitude.

The North Carolina laws describe each of the numbered powers as follows:

Line 1. Real Property Transactions: This line gives your Attorney(s)-in-Fact the authority to lease, purchase, exchange, and acquire, and to agree, bargain, and contract for the lease, purchase, exchange, and acquisition of, and to accept, take, receive, and possess any interest in real property whatsoever, on such terms and conditions, and under such covenants, as your Attorney(s)-in-Fact shall deem proper; and to maintain, repair, improve, manage, insure, rent, lease, sell, convey, subject to liens, mortgage, subject to deeds of trust, and in any way or manner deal with all or any part of any interest in real property whatsoever, that you own at the time of execution or may thereafter acquire, under such terms and conditions, and under such cove-

nants, as your Attorney(s)-in-Fact shall deem proper.

Line 2. Personal Property Transactions: This line gives your Attorney(s)-in-Fact the power to lease, purchase, exchange, and acquire, and to agree, bargain, and contract for the lease, purchase, exchange, and acquisition of, and to accept, take, receive, and possess any personal property whatsoever, tangible or intangible, or interest thereto, on such terms and conditions, and under such covenants, as your Attorney(s)-in-Fact shall deem proper; and to maintain, repair, improve, manage, insure, rent, lease, sell, convey, subject to liens and mortgages, and hypothecate, and in any way or manner deal with all or any part of any personal property whatsoever, tangible or intangible, or any interest therein, that you own at the time of execution or may thereafter acquire, under such terms and conditions, and under such covenants, as your Attorney(s)-in-Fact shall deem proper.

Line 3. Bond, Share and Commodity Transactions: This line enables your Attorney(s)-in-Fact to request, ask, demand, sue for, recover, collect, receive, and hold and possess any bond, share, instrument of similar character, commodity interest, or any instrument with respect thereto together with the interest, dividends, proceeds, or other distributions connected therewith, as now are, or shall hereafter become, owned by, or due, owing payable, or belonging to, you at the time of execution or in which you may thereafter acquire interest, to have, use, and take all lawful means and equitable and legal remedies, procedures, and writs in your name for the collection and recovery thereof, and to adjust, sell, compromise, and agree for the same, and to make, execute, and deliver for you, all endorsements, acquittances, releases, receipts, or other sufficient discharges for the same.

Line 4. Banking Transactions: This line gives your Attorney(s)-in-Fact the power to make, receive, sign, endorse, execute, acknowledge, deliver, and possess checks, drafts, bills of exchange, letters of credit, notes, stock certificates, withdrawal receipts, and deposit instruments relating to accounts or deposits in, or certificates of deposit of, banks, savings and loan, or other institutions or associations for you.

Line 5. Safe Deposits: This line authorizes your Attorney(s)-in-Fact to have free access at any time or times to any safe-deposit box or vault to which you might have access as lessee or owner.

Line 6. Business Operating Transactions: This line allows your Attorney(s)-in-Fact to conduct, engage in, and transact any and all lawful business of whatever nature or kind for you.

Line 7. Insurance Transactions: This line provides your Attorney(s)-in-Fact with authority to exercise or perform any act, power, duty, right, or obligation whatsoever in regard to any contract of life, accident, health, disability, or liability insurance or any combination of such insurance procured by you or on your behalf prior to execution; and to procure new, different, or additional contracts of insurance for you and to designate the beneficiary of any such contract of insurance, provided, however, that the agent himself cannot be such beneficiary unless the agent is your spouse, child, grandchild, parent, brother, or sister.

Line 8. Estate Transactions: This line permits your Attorney(s)-in-Fact to request, ask, demand, sue for, recover, collect, receive, and hold and possess all legacies, bequests, devises, as are owned by, or due, owing, payable, or belonging to, you at the time of execution or in which you may thereafter acquire interest, to have, use, and take all lawful means and equitable and legal remedies, procedures, and writs in your name for the collection and recovery thereof, and to adjust, sell, compromise, and agree for the same, and to make, execute, and deliver for you, all endorsements, acquittances, releases, receipts, or other sufficient discharges for the same.

Line 9. Personal Relationships and Affairs: This line gives your Attorney(s)-in-Fact the power to do all acts necessary for maintaining the customary standard of living of you and your spouse, children, and other dependents; to provide medical, dental, and surgical care, hospitalization, and custodial care for you and your spouse, children, and other dependents; to continue whatever provision has been made by you for you and your spouse, children, and other dependents, with respect to automobiles,

or other means of transportation; to continue whatever charge accounts have been operated by you, for the convenience of you and your spouse, children, and other dependents, to open such new accounts as your Attorney(s)-in-Fact shall think to be desirable for the accomplishment of any of the purposes enumerated in this section, and to pay the items charged on such accounts by any person authorized or permitted by you or your Attorney(s)-in-Fact to make such charges; to continue the discharge of any services or duties assumed by you, to any parent, relative, or friend of yours; to continue payments incidental to the membership or affiliation of you in any church, club, society, order, or other organization, or to continue contributions thereto.

Line 10. Social Security and Unemployment: This line authorizes your Attorney(s)-in-Fact to prepare, execute, and file all social security, unemployment insurance, and information returns required by the laws of the United States, or of any state or subdivision thereof, or of any foreign government.

Line 11. Benefits from Military Service: This line empowers your Attorney(s)-in-Fact to execute vouchers in your name for any and all allowances and reimbursements payable by the United States, or subdivision thereof, to you, arising from or based upon military service and to receive, to endorse, and to collect the proceeds of any check payable to the order of you drawn on the treasurer or other fiscal officer or depository of the United States or subdivision thereof; to take possession and to order the removal and shipment, of any property of yours from any post, warehouse, depot, dock, or other place of storage or safekeeping, either governmental or private, to execute and to deliver any release, voucher, receipt, bill of lading, shipping ticket, certificate, or other instrument that the agent shall think to be desirable or necessary for such purpose; to prepare, to file, and to prosecute your claim to any benefit or assistance, financial or otherwise, to which you are, or you claim to be, entitled, under the provisions of any statute or regulation existing at the creation of the agency or thereafter enacted by the United States or by any state or by any subdivision thereof, or by any foreign government, which benefit or assistance arises from or is based upon military service performed prior to or after execution of this Durable General Power of Attorney.

Line 12. Tax: This line allows your Attorney(s)-in-Fact to prepare, execute, verify, and file in your name and on your behalf any and all types of tax returns, amended returns, declaration of estimated tax, report, protest, application for correction of assessed valuation of real or other property, appeal, brief, claim for refund, or petition, including petition to the Tax Court of the United States, in connection with any tax imposed or proposed to be imposed by any government, or claimed, levied, or assessed by any government, and to pay any such tax and to obtain any extension of time for any of the foregoing; to execute waivers or consents agreeing to a later determination and assessment of taxes than is provided by any statute of limitations; to execute waivers of restriction on the assessment and collection of deficiency in any tax; to execute closing agreements and all other documents, instruments, and papers relating to any tax liability of any sort; to institute and carry on through counsel any proceeding in connection with determining or contesting any such tax or to recover any tax paid or to resist any claim for additional tax on any proposed assessment or levy thereof; and to enter into any agreements or stipulations for compromise or other adjustment or disposition of any tax.

Line 13. Employment of Agents: This line grants to your Attorney(s)-in-Fact the right to employ agents such as legal counsel, accountants, or other professional representation as may be appropriate and to grant such agents such powers of attorney or other appropriate authorization as may be required in connection with such representation or by the Internal Revenue Service or other governmental authority.

Closing Paragraphs: The first full paragraph following the numbered lines gives your Attorney(s)-in-Fact the power to appoint someone else to substitute for him or her. This may be especially important if your chosen Attorney(s)-in-Fact became unable to continue to assist you.

The next line is *crucial* to making your power of attorney *durable,* so that it remains valid at the time you will need it most—during your incapacity.

Finally, you must sign and date the document at the end before a notary. The notary fills in, signs, and seals the bottom portion. A notary is authorized by the state or federal government to administer oaths and attests to the authenticity of signatures.

STATE OF SOUTH CAROLINA)
)
COUNTY OF _____)

POWER OF ATTORNEY

KNOW ALL MEN BY THESE PRESENTS that I, _____
_____
(insert name and address of principal) ("Principal"), a resident of the State and County aforesaid, have made, constituted and appointed and by these presents do make, constitute and appoint _____
_____
(insert name and address of the agent) my true and lawful attorney ("Attorney") for the purposes hereinafter set forth.

Subject to the limitations set forth in this paragraph, I have also made, constituted and appointed and by these presents do make, constitute and appoint as my true and lawful standby attorney ("Standby Attorney") _____
(insert name and address of the agent) for the purposes hereinafter set forth. However, in no event is _____ (Standby Attorney) authorized to act hereunder so long as _____ (Attorney) is living, competent to act and has not resigned nor been removed. A Standby Attorney is subject to removal as provided in Article II, paragraph D, hereof.

ARTICLE I

Empowerment of Attorney

Attorney is authorized in Attorney's absolute discretion from time to time and at any time with respect to my property, real or personal, at any time owned or held by me and without authorization of any court and in addition to any other rights, powers or authority granted by any other provision of this Power of Attorney or by statute or general rules of law, and regardless of whether I am mentally incompetent or physically or mentally disabled or incapable of managing my property and income, with full power of substitution, as follows:

§A. *Powers in General*

To do and perform all and every act, deed, matter and thing whatsoever in and about my estate, property and affairs as fully and effectually to all intents and purposes as I might or could do in my own proper person, if personally present, the specifically enumerated powers described below being in aid and exemplification of the full, complete and general power herein granted and not in limitation or definition thereof.

§B. *Powers Relating to Management of Assets*

1. To buy, receive, lease as lessor, accept or otherwise acquire; to sell, convey, mortgage, grant options upon, hypothecate, pledge, transfer, exchange, quitclaim or otherwise encumber or dispose of; or to contract or agree for the acquisition, disposal or encumbrance of any property whatsoever or any custody, possession, interest or right therein, for cash or credit and upon such terms, considerations and conditions as Attorney shall think proper, and no person dealing with Attorney shall be bound to see to the application of any monies paid;

2. To take, hold, possess, invest or otherwise manage any or all of my property or any interest therein; to eject, remove or relieve tenants or other persons from, and recover possession of, such property by all lawful means; and to maintain, protect, preserve, insure, remove, store, transport, repair, build on, raze, rebuild, alter, modify or improve the same or any part thereof and/or to lease any property, real or personal for me or my benefit, as lessee, with or without option to renew; to collect, receive and receipt for rents, issues and profits of my property;

3. To make, endorse, accept, receive, sign, seal, execute, acknowledge and deliver deeds, assignments, agreements, certificates, endorsements, hypothecations, checks, notes, mortgages,

vouchers, receipts, consents, waivers, releases, undertakings, satisfactions, acknowledgements and such other documents or instruments in writing of whatever kind and nature as may be necessary, convenient or proper in the premises;

4.   To subdivide, develop or dedicate real property to public use or to make or obtain the vacation of plats and adjust boundaries, to adjust differences in valuation on exchange or partition by giving or receiving consideration, and to dedicate easements to public use without consideration;

5.   To invest and reinvest all or any part of my property in any property and undivided interest in property, wherever located, including bonds, debentures, notes, secured or unsecured, stocks of corporations regardless of class, interest in limited partnerships, real estate or any interest in real estate whether or not productive at the time of investment, interest in trusts, investment trusts, whether of the open and/or closed fund types and participation in common, collective or pooled trust funds or annuity contracts without being limited by any statute or rule of law concerning investments by fiduciaries;

6.   To continue and operate any business owned by me and to do any and all things deemed needful or appropriate by Attorney, including the power to incorporate the business and to put additional capital into the business, for such time as Attorney shall deem advisable, without liability for loss resulting from the continuance or operation of the business except for Attorney's own negligence; and to close out, liquidate or sell the business at such time and upon such terms as Attorney shall deem best;

7.   To transfer all of my stock and/or securities to my Attorney, as agent (with the beneficial ownership thereof remaining in me), if necessary or convenient, in order to exercise the powers with respect to such stock and/or securities granted herein;

8.   To sell or exercise stock subscription or conversion rights;

9.   To refrain from voting or to vote shares of stock owned by me at shareholder's meetings in person or by special, limited or general proxy and in general to exercise all the rights, powers and privileges of an owner in respect to any securities constituting my property;

10.   To participate in any plan of reorganization or consolidation or merger involving any company or companies with respect to stock or other securities which I own and to deposit such stock or other securities under any plan or reorganization or with any protective committee and to delegate to such committee discretionary power with relation thereto, to pay a proportionate part of the expenses of such committee and any assessments levied under any such plan, to accept and retain new securities received by Attorney pursuant to any such plan, to exercise all conversion, subscription, voting and other rights, of whatsoever nature pertaining to such property, and to pay any amount or amounts of money that Attorney may deem advisable in connection therewith;

11.   To institute, prosecute, defend, abandon, compromise, arbitrate and dispose of legal, equitable or administrative hearings, actions, suits, attachments, arrests, distresses or other proceedings or otherwise engage in litigation involving me, my property or any interest of mine;

12.   To deal with Attorney in Attorney's individual or any fiduciary capacity, in buying and selling assets, in lending and borrowing money, and in all other transactions, irrespective of the occupancy by the same person of dual positions;

13.   To insure my property against damage or loss and Attorney against liability with respect to third persons.

§C. *Powers Relating to Custody of Person*

1.   In general, and in addition to all the specific acts in this section enumerated, to do any other act or acts, which I can do through an agent, for the welfare of my spouse, children and/or

dependents or for the preservation and maintenance of my other personal relationships to parents, relatives, friends and organizations;

2.　To do all acts necessary for maintaining the customary standard of living of my spouse, children and/or dependents of mine, including by way of illustration and not by way of restriction, power to provide living quarters by purchase, lease or by other contract, or by payment of the operating costs, including interest, amortization payments, repairs and taxes, of premises owned by me and occupied by my family and/or dependents, to provide usual educational facilities, and to provide funds for all the current living costs of my spouse, children and/or dependents of mine, including food and incidentals, and if necessary to make all necessary arrangements, contractual or otherwise, for me at any hospital, nursing home, convalescent home or similar establishment;

3.　To continue whatever provision has been made by me, prior to the creation of this power or thereafter, for my spouse, children and/or dependents, with respect to automobiles, or other means of transportation, including by way of illustration but not by way of restriction, power to license, to insure and to replace any automobiles owned by me and customarily used by my spouse, children and/or dependents; to apply for a Certificate of Title upon, and endorse and transfer title thereto, any automobile, truck pickup, van, motorcycle or other motor vehicle and to represent in such transfer assignment that the title to said motor vehicle is free and clear of all liens and encumbrances except those specifically set forth in such transfer assignment;

4.　To continue whatever charge accounts have been operated by me prior to the creation of this power or thereafter, for the convenience of my spouse, children and/or dependents, to open such new accounts as Attorney shall think to be desirable for the accomplishment of any of the purposes enumerated in this section, and to pay the items charged on such accounts by any person authorized or permitted by me to make such charges prior to the creation of the power;

5.　To continue the discharge of any services or duties assumed by me prior to the creation of this power or thereafter, to any parent, relative or friend of mine;

6.　To supervise, compromise, enforce, arbitrate, defend or settle any claim by or against me arising out of property damages or personal injuries suffered by or caused by me, or under such circumstances that the loss resulting therefrom will, or may, fall on me; or to intervene in any action or proceeding relating thereto;

7.　To continue payments incidental to my membership or affiliation in any church, club, society, order or other organization or to continue contributions thereto;

8.　To demand, to receive, to obtain by action, proceeding or otherwise any money or other thing of value to which I am or may become or may claim to be entitled as salary, wages, commissions or other distributions upon any stock, or as interest or principal upon any indebtedness, or any periodic distribution of profits from any partnership or business in which I have or claim an interest, and to endorse, collect or otherwise realize upon any instrument for the payment so received;

9.　To prepare, to execute and to file all joint or separate tax, social security, unemployment insurance and information returns for any years required by the laws of the United States, or of any state or subdivision thereof, or of any foreign government, to prepare, to execute and to file all other papers and instruments which Attorney shall think to be desirable or necessary for safeguarding me against excess or illegal taxation or against penalties imposed for claimed violation of any law or other governmental regulation, and to pay, to compromise, or to contest or to apply for refunds in connection with any taxes or assessments for which I am or may be liable, to consent to any gift for the gift tax purposes and to utilize any gift-splitting provision, or to make any tax election;

10.　To execute, to acknowledge, to verify, to seal, to file and to deliver any application, consent, petition, notice, release, waiver, agreement or other instrument which Attorney may think useful for the accomplishment of any of the purposes enumerated in this section;

11.   To hire, to discharge and to compensate any attorney, accountant, expert witness or other assistant(s) where Attorney shall think such action to be desirable for the proper execution by Attorney of any of the powers described in this section, and for the keeping of needed records thereof;

12.   To employ and compensate medical personnel including physicians, surgeons, dentists, medical specialists, nurses and paramedical assistants deemed by Attorney needful for the proper care, custody and control of my person and to do so without liability for any neglect, omission, misconduct or fault of any such physician or other medical personnel, provided such physician or other medical personnel were selected and retained with reasonable care, and to dismiss any such persons at any time, with or without cause;

13.   To authorize any and all kinds of medical procedures and treatment including but not limited to medication, therapy, surgical procedures and dental care, and to consent to all such treatment and medical procedures where such consent is required; to obtain the use of medical equipment, devices or other equipment and devices deemed by Attorney needful for proper care, custody and control of my person and to do so without liability for any neglect, omission, misconduct or fault with respect to such medical treatment or other matters authorized herein;

14.   To apply for, elect, receive, deposit and utilize on my behalf all benefits payable by any governmental body or agency, state, federal, county, city or other and to obtain, make claim upon, collect and dispose of insurance and insurance proceeds for my care, custody and control;

15.   To house (or provide for housing), support and maintain any animals which I own and to contract for and pay the expenses of proper veterinary care and treatment for such animals, or if the care and maintenance of such animals shall become unreasonably expensive in Attorney's opinion to dispose of such animals;

16.   To deposit in my name and for my account, with any bank, banker or trust company or any building or savings and loan association or any other banking or similar institution, all monies to which I am entitled or which may come into Attorney's hands as such attorney-in-fact, and all bills of exchange, drafts, checks, promissory notes and other securities for money payable belonging to me, and for that purpose to sign my name and endorse each and every such instrument for deposit or collection; and from time to time, or at any time, to withdraw any or all monies deposited to my credit at any bank, banker or trust company or any building or savings and loan association or any other banking or similar institution having monies belonging to me, and, in connection therewith, to draw checks or to make withdrawals in my name; to make, do, execute, acknowledge and deliver, for and upon my behalf and in my name, all such checks, notes and contracts;

17.   To endorse, receive, deposit and/or collect checks payable to my order drawn on the Treasurer or other fiscal officer or depository of the United States, or any sovereign state or authority, or any political subdivision or instrumentality thereof, or any private person, firm, corporation or partnership;

18.   To have access at any time or times to any safe deposit box rented by me, wheresoever located, and to remove all or any part of the contents thereof, and to surrender or relinquish said safe deposit box, and any institution in which any such safe deposit box may be located shall not incur any liability to me or my estate as a result of permitting Attorney to exercise this power;

19.   To borrow money and to encumber, mortgage or pledge any and all of my property in connection with the exercise of any power vested in Attorney;

20. To purchase for my benefit and in my behalf United States Government bonds redeemable at par in payment of United States estate taxes imposed at my death upon my estate;

21. To make advance arrangements for funeral services, including, but not limited to, purchase of a burial plot and marker and such other and related arrangements for services, flowers, ministerial services, transportation and other necessary, related, convenient or appropriate goods and services as my Attorney shall deem advisable or appropriate under the circumstances.

ARTICLE II

Termination, Amendment, Resignation and Removal

§A. *Power Not Affected by Principal's Incapacity*

This Power of Attorney shall not be affected by physical disability or mental incompetence of the principal which renders the principal incapable of managing his own estate. It is my intent that the authority conferred herein shall be exercisable notwithstanding my physical disability or mental incompetence.

§B. *Termination and Amendment*

This Power of Attorney shall remain in full force and effect until the earlier of the following events: (i) Attorney has resigned as provided herein; (ii) I have revoked this Power of Attorney by written instrument recorded in the public records of the county aforesaid; or (iii) a committee shall have been appointed for me by a court of competent jurisdiction. This Power of Attorney may be amended by me at any time and from time to time but such amendment shall not be effective as to third persons dealing with Attorney without notice of such amendment unless such amendment shall have been recorded in the public records of the county aforesaid.

§C. *Resignation*

In the event that Attorney shall become unable or unwilling to serve or continue to serve, then Attorney may resign by delivering to me in writing a copy of his resignation and recording the original in the public records of the county aforesaid. Upon such resignation and recording, Attorney shall thereupon be divested of all authority under this Power of Attorney.

§D. *Removal*

Any person named herein as Attorney may be removed by written instrument executed by me and recorded in the public records of the county aforesaid.

ARTICLE III

Incidental Powers and Binding Effect

In connection with the exercise of the powers herein described, Attorney is fully authorized and empowered to perform any other acts or things necessary, appropriate, or incidental thereto, with the same validity and effect as if I were personally present, competent and personally exercised the powers myself. All acts lawfully done by Attorney hereunder during any period of my disability or mental incompetence shall have the same effect and inure to the benefit of and bind me and my heirs, devises, legatees and personal representatives as if I were mentally competent and not disabled. The powers herein conferred may be exercised by Attorney alone and the signature or act of Attorney on my behalf may be accepted by third persons as fully authorized by me and with the same force and effect as if done under my hand and seal and as if I were present in person, acting on my own behalf and competent. No person who may act in reliance upon the representations of Attorney for the scope of authority granted to Attorney shall incur any liability to me or to my estate as a result of permitting Attorney to exercise any power, nor shall any person dealing with Attorney be responsible to determine or insure the proper application of funds or property.

ARTICLE IV
Miscellaneous

§A. *Exculpation*

Attorney, Attorney's heirs, successors and assigns are hereby released and forever discharged from any and all liability upon any claim or demand of any nature whatsoever by me, my heirs or assigns, the beneficiaries under my Will or under any trust which I have created or shall hereafter create or any person whomsoever on account of any failure to act as Attorney pursuant to this Power of Attorney.

§B. *Definitions*

Whenever the word "Attorney" or "Principal" or any modifying or substituted pronoun therefor is used in this Power of Attorney, such words and respective pronouns shall be held and taken to include both the singular and the plural, the masculine, feminine and neuter gender thereof.

§C. *Severability*

If any part of any provision of this Power of Attorney shall be invalid or unenforceable under applicable law, said part shall be ineffective to the extent of such invalidity only, without in any way affecting the remaining parts of said provision or the remaining provisions of this Power of Attorney.

§D. *Compensation*

Attorney shall be entitled to reimbursement for all reasonable costs and expenses actually incurred and paid by Attorney on my behalf pursuant to any provision of this Power of Attorney.

§E. *Restrictions*

Notwithstanding any provision herein to the contrary, Attorney shall not satisfy the legal obligations of Attorney out of any property subject to this Power of Attorney, nor may Attorney exercise this power in favor of Attorney, Attorney's estate, Attorney's creditors or the creditors of Attorney's estate.

§F. *Reservations*

Notwithstanding any provision hereto to the contrary, Attorney shall have no power or authority whatsoever with respect to (a) any policy of insurance owned by me on the life of Attorney, and (b) any trust created by Attorney as to which I am a trustee.

IN WITNESS WHEREOF, as Principal, I have executed this Power of Attorney as of this _____ day of _____, 19___, in multiple counter-part originals and I have directed that photographic copies of this Power be made which shall have the same force and effect as an original.

_____ (Seal)
                    Principal

STATE OF SOUTH CAROLINA)
)   **ATTESTATION**
COUNTY OF _____)

       The foregoing Power of Attorney was made this _____ day of _____, 19___, signed, sealed, published and declared by the Principal as the Principal's appointment and empowerment of an attorney-in-fact, in the presence of us who at the Principal's request and in the Principal's presence and in the presence of each other, have hereunto subscribed our names as witnesses hereto.

_____ of

_____

_____ of

_____

_____ of

_____

STATE OF SOUTH CAROLINA)
)   **PROBATE**
COUNTY OF _____)

       Personally appeared deponent and made oath that deponent saw the within named Principal sign, seal and as the Principal's act and deed deliver the within Power of Attorney and that deponent, with the other witnesses whose names are subscribed above, witnessed the execution thereof.

_____

SWORN to before me this _____ day
of _____, 19___.

_____(Seal)
Notary Public for South Carolina
My Commission Expires: _____

Durable Power of Attorney
(South Carolina)

Instructions/Explanation

The explanations that follow should provide you with a clear understanding of the terms used in the following Durable Power of Attorney.

Introduction: At the top left, you will see the words "State of South Carolina" and "County of _____." Fill in the name of your county. Use a pen, not a pencil.

Below that, fill in your name and address (you are the "principal"—the person making the Durable Power of Attorney).

On the next lines, fill in the name and address of the person to whom you are giving the Durable Power of Attorney (called the "Agent" or "Attorney").

Article I: The following lettered clauses specify broad powers providing your Attorney with wide latitude to manage your financial affairs. Powers are separately enumerated to avoid any questions about whether you intended to authorize your Attorney to undertake specific actions on your behalf. In addition, the introductory paragraph to Article I indicates that your Durable Power of Attorney can be used whether you are competent or incompetent.

Article II: Section A is *crucial* to making your power of attorney *durable,* so that it remains valid at the time you will need it most—during your incapacity.

Section B specifies that your Durable Power of Attorney will remain in effect until your Attorney resigns, you revoke it in a writing that is properly recorded, or a committee is appointed for you by a court. Amendments also are not effective unless they are properly recorded.

Sections C and D set forth the procedure for withdrawal or removal of your Attorney.

Article III: The first sentence is a general, catch-all provision authorizing your Attorney to do anything you could do.

Article III also provides assurance to third parties, such as banks and insurance companies, that they may rely on actions taken by your Attorney under the Durable Power of Attorney.

Article IV: Section A says that your Attorney will not be liable to anyone for failing to act as Attorney under the Durable Power of Attorney.

Section B is just a definitional section.

Section C says that if any part of the Durable Power of Attorney is held by a court to be invalid, the rest of the document would remain valid.

Section D provides reimbursement for your Attorney's costs.

Section E makes it clear that your Attorney is to take action under the Durable Power of Attorney only on your behalf, not on his/her own behalf.

Section F says that your Attorney cannot take actions concerning insurance that you own on the life of the Attorney or a trust created by the Attorney for which you are a trustee.

Finally, sign and date the document at the end before three witnesses and a notary, who must sign and date the document too. The witnesses should also provide their addresses.

STATUTORY SHORT FORM
DURABLE GENERAL POWER OF ATTORNEY

NOTICE: The powers granted by this document are broad and sweeping. They are defined in New York General Obligations Law, Article 5, Title 15, Sections 5–1502A through 5–1503, which expressly permits the use of any other or different form of power of attorney desired by the parties concerned.

Know All Men by These Presents, which are intended to constitute a GENERAL POWER OF ATTORNEY pursuant to Article 5, Title 15 of the New York General Obligations Law:

That I, _____ ,

_____

(insert name and address of the principal)

do hereby appoint _____

_____

_____ ,

(insert name and address of the agent, or
each agent, if more than one is designated)

my attorney(s)-in-fact TO ACT _____ .

(If more than one agent is designated and the principal wishes each agent alone to be able to exercise the power conferred, insert in this blank the word 'severally'. Failure to make any insertion or the insertion of the word 'jointly' will require the agents to act jointly.)

In my name, place and stead in any way which I myself could do, if I were personally present, with respect to the following matters as each of them is defined in Title 15 of Article 5 of the New York General Obligations Law to the extent that I am permitted by law to act through an agent:

(Strike out and initial in the opposite box any one or more of the subdivisions as to which the principal does NOT desire to give the agent authority. Such elimination of any one or more of subdivisions (A) to (L), inclusive, shall automatically constitute an elimination also of subdivision (M).)

To strike out any subdivision the principal must draw a line through the text of that subdivision AND write his initials in the box opposite.

(A)	real estate transactions;	( )
(B)	chattel and goods transactions;	( )
(C)	bond, share and commodity transactions;	( )
(D)	banking transactions;	( )
(E)	business operating transactions;	( )
(F)	insurance transactions;	( )
(G)	estate transactions;	( )
(H)	claims and litigation;	( )
(I)	personal relationships and affairs;	( )
(J)	benefits from military service;	( )

(K)	records, reports and statements;	( )
(L)	full and unqualified authority to my attorney(s)-in-fact to delegate any or all of the foregoing powers to any person or persons whom my attorney(s)-in-fact shall select;	( )
(M)	all other matters;	( )

_____

_____

_____

_____

_____

_____

(Special provisions and limitations may be included in the statutory short form power of attorney only if they conform to the requirements of section 5–1503 of the New York General Obligations Law.)

This power of attorney shall not be affected by the subsequent disability or incompetence of the principal.

TO INDUCE ANY THIRD PARTY TO ACT HEREUNDER, I HEREBY AGREE THAT ANY THIRD PARTY RECEIVING A DULY EXECUTED COPY OR FACSIMILE OF THIS INSTRUMENT MAY ACT HEREUNDER, AND THAT REVOCATION OR TERMINATION HEREOF SHALL BE INEFFECTIVE AS TO SUCH THIRD PARTY UNLESS AND UNTIL ACTUAL NOTICE OR KNOWLEDGE OF SUCH REVOCATION OR TERMINATION SHALL HAVE BEEN RECEIVED BY SUCH THIRD PARTY, AND I FOR MYSELF AND FOR MY HEIRS, EXECUTORS, LEGAL REPRESENTATIVES AND ASSIGNS, HEREBY AGREE TO INDEMNIFY AND HOLD HARMLESS ANY SUCH THIRD PARTY FROM AND AGAINST ANY AND ALL CLAIMS THAT MAY ARISE AGAINST SUCH THIRD PARTY BY REASON OF SUCH THIRD PARTY HAVING RELIED ON THE PROVISIONS OF THIS INSTRUMENT.

In Witness Whereof, I have hereunto signed my name and affixed my seal this ____ day of _____, 19___.

_____ (Seal)

(Signature of Principal)

Specimen Signature of Attorney(s)-in-Fact:

_____

_____

Signed in the presence of:

_____

_____

_____
Witness

_____
Witness

2

CERTIFICATE OF NOTARY

STATE OF NEW YORK   )

) SS:

COUNTY OF _____)

       On the _____ day of _____, 19___, before me personally came _____, whose identity is well known to me to be the individual described in and who executed the foregoing instrument, and (he)(she) acknowledged to me that (he)(she) executed the same.

                                              _____

                                             Notary Public

My commission expires:

_____

Statutory Short Form
Durable General Power of Attorney
(New York)

Instructions/Explanation

The explanations that follow should provide you with a clear understanding of the terms used in the Statutory Short Form Durable General Power of Attorney.

Notice: The notice confirms what the book has already stated: the powers given to your Attorney(s)-in-Fact are broad.

Introduction: On the first blank line, fill in your name and address (you are the "principal"—the person making the Durable General Power of Attorney).

On the next lines, fill in the name(s) and address(es) of the person(s) to whom you are giving the Durable General Power of Attorney (called the "agent(s)" or "attorney(s)-in-fact").

If you have decided to name more than one Attorney-in-Fact, you should fill in the next blank either with the word "severally" or "jointly." "Severally" means that either of your Attorneys-in-Fact on his/her own will be able to exercise the powers provided in the Durable General Power of Attorney; "jointly" means that your Attorneys-in-Fact must act together to use your Durable General Power of Attorney.

The following lettered clauses specify broad powers providing your Attorney(s)-in-Fact with wide latitude to manage your affairs. Powers are separately enumerated to avoid any questions about whether you intended to authorize your Attorney(s)-in-Fact to undertake specific actions on your behalf. If you choose not to give all these powers to your Attorney(s)-in-Fact, you must draw a line through the power(s) which you want to exclude *and* initial inside the parentheses after such excluded power(s).

Clause A: This clause gives your Attorney(s)-in-Fact broad authority to mortgage, sell, buy, accept, manage, lease, and/or otherwise deal with real estate, including your home.

Clause B: This clause permits your Attorney(s)-in-Fact broad authority to buy, sell, manage, receive, mortgage, lease, and/or otherwise handle transactions involving items of personal property.

Clause C: This clause lets your Attorney(s)-in-Fact invest in securities on your behalf and to manage, receive, sell, mortgage, and/or otherwise handle securities for you. This is broad enough to allow your Attorney(s)-in-Fact even to vote at stockholders meetings.

Clause D: This clause authorizes your Attorney(s)-in-Fact to handle banking transactions, including to open and manage accounts, CDs, and other instruments in financial institutions, to sign checks, to make withdrawals, and to have access to your safe-deposit box.

Clause E: This clause allows your Attorney(s)-in-Fact to engage in any business transactions for you.

Clause F: This clause authorizes your Attorney(s)-in-Fact to handle insurance matters for you, including obtaining, managing, maintaining, or terminating insurance, paying premiums, and obtaining benefits for you.

Clause G: This clause permits your Attorney(s)-in-Fact to act for you with respect to estate matters, including receiving inheritances and participating in the administration of estates.

Clause H: This clause gives your Attorney(s)-in-Fact the right to handle claims and litigation for you, including to bring a lawsuit for you, to defend you against claims, and to settle disputes for you.

Clause I: This clause authorizes your Attorney(s)-in-Fact to handle your personal affairs, to take steps to provide for the support and welfare of your family, and to maintain your relationships with family, friends, and organizations.

Clause J: This clause enables your Attorney(s)-in-Fact to handle any matters you may have with the military, including making and receiving proceeds of any claims and maximizing benefits from military service.

Clause K: This clause empowers your Attorney(s)-in-Fact to make, execute, file and store and keep records, reports, and statements, including tax returns, for you.

Clause L: This clause allows your Attorney(s)-in-Fact to delegate his/her powers to someone else.

Clause M: This clause is a general, catch-all authorizing your Attorney(s)-in-Fact to do anything you could do.

On the lines that follow, you could add other provisions or limitations, but if you try to do this, you'd better make sure your additions or changes comply with the law.

The next sentence is *crucial* to making your power of attorney *durable*, so that it remains valid at the time you will need it most—during your incapacity.

Some banks and insurance companies have traditionally been unwilling to accept or act on any preprinted power of attorney form that they did not prepare themselves. That last full paragraph printed in all capital letters attempts to deal with this problem. That paragraph will protect third parties relying on the Durable General Power of Attorney and, it is hoped, encourage them to accept this form. However, since there can be no assurance that this will work, you should contact your bank and insurance company to discuss their forms and procedures.

Finally, sign and date the document at the end before two witnesses and a notary. Have the Attorney(s)-in-Fact sign his or her name under yours. The notary fills in and signs the bottom portion. A notary is authorized by the state or federal government to administer oaths and attest to the authenticity of signatures.

STATUTORY SHORT FORM POWER OF ATTORNEY
(California Civil Code Section 2450)

WARNING. UNLESS YOU LIMIT THE POWER IN THIS DOCUMENT, THIS DOCUMENT GIVES YOUR AGENT THE POWER TO ACT FOR YOU IN ANY WAY YOU COULD ACT FOR YOURSELF. FOR EXAMPLE, YOUR AGENT CAN:

BUY, SELL, AND MANAGE REAL AND PERSONAL PROPERTY FOR YOU. THIS MEANS THAT YOUR AGENT CAN SELL YOUR HOME, YOUR SECURITIES, AND YOUR OTHER PROPERTY.

DEPOSIT AND WITHDRAW MONEY FROM YOUR CHECKING AND SAVINGS ACCOUNTS.

BORROW MONEY USING YOUR PROPERTY AS SECURITY FOR THE LOAN.

PUT THINGS IN AND TAKE THINGS OUT OF YOUR SAFETY DEPOSIT BOX.

OPERATE YOUR BUSINESS FOR YOU.

PREPARE AND FILE TAX RETURNS FOR YOU AND ACT FOR YOU IN TAX MATTERS.

ESTABLISH TRUSTS FOR YOU AND TAKE OTHER ACTIONS FOR YOU IN CONNECTION WITH PROBATE AND ESTATE PLANNING MATTERS.

PROVIDE FOR THE SUPPORT AND WELFARE OF YOUR SPOUSE, CHILDREN, AND DEPENDENTS.

CONTINUE PAYMENTS TO THE CHURCH AND OTHER ORGANIZATIONS OF WHICH YOU ARE A MEMBER AND MAKE GIFTS TO YOUR SPOUSE, DESCENDANTS, AND CHARITIES.

THIS DOCUMENT DOES NOT AUTHORIZE YOUR AGENT TO MAKE MEDICAL AND OTHER HEALTH CARE DECISIONS FOR YOU. YOU CAN DESIGNATE AN AGENT TO MAKE HEALTH CARE DECISIONS FOR YOU ONLY BY A SEPARATE DOCUMENT.

IT MAY BE IN YOUR BEST INTEREST TO CONSULT WITH A CALIFORNIA LAWYER BECAUSE THE POWERS GRANTED BY THIS DOCUMENT ARE BROAD AND SWEEPING. THEY ARE DEFINED IN SECTIONS 2460 TO 2473, INCLUSIVE, OF THE CALIFORNIA CIVIL CODE.

THE POWERS GRANTED BY THIS DOCUMENT WILL EXIST FOR AN INDEFINITE PERIOD OF TIME UNLESS YOU LIMIT THEIR DURATION IN THIS DOCUMENT. THESE POWERS WILL CONTINUE TO EXIST NOTWITHSTANDING YOUR SUBSEQUENT DISABILITY OR INCAPACITY UNLESS YOU INDICATE OTHERWISE IN THIS DOCUMENT.

YOU CAN ELIMINATE POWERS OF YOUR AGENT BY CROSSING OUT ANY ONE OR MORE OF THE POWERS LISTED IN PARAGRAPH 3 OF THIS FORM. YOU CAN WRITE OTHER LIMITATIONS AND SPECIAL PROVISIONS IN PARAGRAPH 4 OF THIS FORM. HOWEVER, IF YOU DO NOT WANT TO GRANT YOUR AGENT THE POWER TO ACT FOR YOU IN ANY WAY YOU COULD ACT FOR YOURSELF, IT MAY BE IN YOUR BEST INTEREST TO CONSULT WITH A LAWYER INSTEAD OF USING THIS FORM.

THIS DOCUMENT MUST BE SIGNED BY TWO WITNESSES AND BE NOTARIZED TO BE VALID.

YOU HAVE THE RIGHT TO REVOKE OR TERMINATE THIS POWER OF ATTORNEY.

YOU ARE NOT REQUIRED TO USE THIS FORM; YOU MAY USE A DIFFERENT POWER OF ATTORNEY IF THAT IS DESIRED BY THE PARTIES CONCERNED.

IF THERE IS ANYTHING ABOUT THIS FORM THAT YOU DO NOT UNDERSTAND, YOU SHOULD ASK A LAWYER TO EXPLAIN IT TO YOU.

1. DESIGNATION OF AGENT.

I, _____,

(Insert your name and address)

do hereby appoint_____

_____

(Insert name and address of your agent, or each agent
if you want to designate more than one)

as my attorney(s)-in-fact (agent) to act for me and in my name as authorized in this document.

2. CREATION OF DURABLE POWER OF ATTORNEY. By this document I intend to create a general power of attorney under Sections 2450 to 2473, inclusive, of the California Civil Code. Subject to any limitations in this document, this power of attorney is a durable power of attorney and shall not be affected by my subsequent incapacity.

(If you want this power of attorney to terminate automatically when you lack capacity, you must so state in paragraph 4 ("Special Provisions and Limitations") below.)

3. STATEMENT OF AUTHORITY GRANTED. Subject to any limitations in this document, I hereby grant to my agent(s) full power and authority to act for me and in my name in any way which I myself could act if I were personally present and able to act, with respect to the following matters as each of them is defined in Chapter 3 (commencing with Section 2450) of Title 9 of Part 4 of Division 3 of the California Civil Code to the extent that I am permitted by law to act through an agent:

      (1)   Real estate transactions.

      (2)   Tangible personal property transactions.

      (3)   Bond, share and commodity transactions.

      (4)   Financial institution transactions.

      (5)   Business operating transactions.

      (6)   Insurance transactions.

      (7)   Retirement plan transactions.

      (8)   Estate transactions.

      (9)   Claims and litigation.

     (10)   Tax matters.

     (11)   Personal relationships and affairs.

     (12)   Benefits from military service.

(13)   Records, reports, and statements.

(14)   Full and unqualified authority to my agent(s) to delegate any or all of the foregoing powers to any person or persons whom my agent(s) shall select.

(15)   All other matters.

(Strike out any one or more of the items above to which you do NOT desire to give your agent authority. Such elimination of any one or more of items (1) to (14), inclusive, automatically constitutes an elimination of item (15). TO STRIKE OUT AN ITEM, YOU MUST DRAW A LINE THROUGH THE TEXT OF THAT ITEM.)

4.   SPECIAL PROVISIONS AND LIMITATIONS. In exercising the authority under this power of attorney, my agent(s) is subject to the following special provisions and limitations:

_____

_____

_____

_____

(Special provisions and limitations may be included in the statutory short form power of attorney only if they conform to the requirements of Section 2455 of the California Civil Code.)

5.   EXERCISE OF POWER OF ATTORNEY WHERE MORE THAN ONE AGENT DESIGNATED. If I have designated more than one agent, the agents are to act _____
_____.

(If you designate more than one agent and wish each agent alone to be able to exercise this power, insert in this blank the word "severally." Failure to make an insertion or the insertion of the word "jointly" will require that the agents act jointly.)

6.   DURATION.

(The powers granted by this document will exist for an indefinite period of time unless you limit their duration below.)

This power of attorney expires on _____.

(Fill in this space ONLY if you want the authority
of your agent to terminate before your death.)

7.   NOMINATION OF CONSERVATOR OF ESTATE.

(A conservator of the estate may be appointed for you if a court decides that one should be appointed. The conservator is responsible for the management of your financial affairs and your property. You are not required to nominate a conservator but you may do so. The court will appoint the person you nominate unless that would be contrary to your best interests. You may, but are not required to, nominate as your conservator the same person you named in paragraph 1 as your agent. You may nominate a person as your conservator by completing the space below.)

If a conservator of the estate is to be appointed for me, I nominate the following person to serve as conservator of the estate _____

_____

(Insert name and address of person nominated as conservator of the estate)

DATE AND SIGNATURE OF PRINCIPAL
(YOU MUST DATE AND SIGN THIS POWER OF ATTORNEY)

I sign my name to this Statutory Short Form Power of Attorney on _____
(Date) at _____(City), _____(State).

_____
(You sign here)

(THIS POWER OF ATTORNEY WILL NOT BE VALID UNLESS IT IS BOTH (1) SIGNED BY TWO ADULT WITNESSES WHO ARE PRESENT WHEN YOU SIGN OR ACKNOWLEDGE YOUR SIGNATURE AND (2) ACKNOWLEDGED BEFORE A NOTARY PUBLIC IN CALIFORNIA.)

STATEMENT OF WITNESSES

(READ CAREFULLY BEFORE SIGNING. You can sign as a witness only if you personally know the principal or the identity of the principal is proved to you by convincing evidence.)

(To have convincing evidence of the identity of the principal, you must be presented with and reasonably rely on any one or more of the following:

(1)   An identification card or driver's license issued by the California Department of Motor Vehicles that is current or has been issued within five years.

(2)   A passport issued by the Department of State of the United States that is current or has been issued within five years.

(3)   Any of the following documents if the document is current or has been issued within five years and contains a photograph and description of the person named on it, is signed by the person, and bears a serial or other identifying number:

(a)   A passport issued by a foreign government that has been stamped by the United States Immigration and Naturalization Service.

(b)   A driver's license issued by a state other than California or by a Canadian or Mexican public agency authorized to issue drivers' licenses.

(c)   An identification card issued by any branch of the armed forces of the United States.)

(Other kinds of proof of identity are not allowed.)

I declare under penalty of perjury under the laws of California that the person who signed or acknowledged this document is personally known to me (or proved to me on the basis of convincing evidence) to be the principal, that the principal signed or acknowledged this power of attorney in my presence, and that the principal appears to be of sound mind and under no duress, fraud, or undue influence.

Signature:_____   Residence Address:_____

Print Name:_____   _____

Date:_____   _____

Signature:_____   Residence Address:_____

Print Name:_____   _____

Date:_____   _____

CERTIFICATE OF ACKNOWLEDGEMENT OF NOTARY PUBLIC

STATE OF CALIFORNIA   )
) SS:

COUNTY OF _____)

On this _____ day of _____, in the year _____, before me,

_____
(Insert name of notary public)

personally appeared _____,
(Insert name of principal)

personally known to me (or proved to me on the basis of satisfactory evidence) to be the person whose name is subscribed to this instrument, and acknowledged that he or she executed it.

NOTARY SEAL

_____
Signature of Notary Public

My commission expires:

_____

Statutory Short Form Power of Attorney
(California)

Instructions/Explanation

The explanations that follow should provide you with a clear understanding of the terms used in the Statutory Short Form Power of Attorney.

Notice: The notice confirms what the book has already stated: the powers given to your Attorney(s)-in-Fact (Agent(s)) are broad. Read the Notice carefully; it provides a good description of the power of attorney.

Paragraph 1: On the first blank line, fill in your name and address.

On the next lines, fill in the name(s) and address(es) of the person(s) to whom you are giving the Statutory Short Form Power of Attorney (called the "Agent(s)" or "Attorney(s)-in-Fact").

Paragraph 2: This paragraph is *crucial* to making your power of attorney *durable,* so that it remains valid at the time you will need it most—during your incapacity.

Paragraph 3: The following numbered clauses specify broad powers providing your Attorney(s)-in-Fact with wide latitude to manage your affairs. Powers are separately enumerated to avoid any questions about whether you intended to authorize your Attorney(s)-in-Fact to undertake specific actions on your behalf. If you choose not to give all these powers to your Attorney(s)-in-Fact, you must draw a line through the powers that you want to exclude.

Line 1: This line gives your Attorney(s)-in-Fact broad authority to mortgage, sell, buy, accept, manage, lease, and/or otherwise deal with real estate, including your home.

Line 2: This line permits your Attorney(s)-in-Fact broad authority to buy, sell, manage, receive, mortgage, lease, and/or otherwise handle transactions involving items of personal property.

Line 3: This line lets your Attorney(s)-in-Fact invest in securities on your behalf and manage, receive, sell, mortgage, and/or otherwise handle securities for you. This is broad enough to allow your Attorney(s)-in-Fact even to vote at stockholders meetings.

Line 4: This line authorizes your Attorney(s)-in-Fact to handle banking transactions, including to open and manage accounts, CDs and other instruments in financial institutions, to sign checks, to make withdrawals, and to have access to your safe-deposit box.

Line 5: This line allows your Attorney(s)-in-Fact to engage in any business transactions for you.

Line 6: This line authorizes your Attorney(s)-in-Fact to handle any insurance matters for you, including obtaining, managing, maintaining, or terminating insurance, paying premiums, and obtaining benefits for you.

Line 7: This line allows your Attorney(s)-in-Fact to handle retirement plan transactions for you, including selecting payment options, making or changing beneficiary designations, making contributions and rollovers, and borrowing from retirement plans.

Line 8: This line permits your Attorney(s)-in-Fact to act for you with respect to estate matters, including establishing trusts, receiving inheritances, and participating in the administration of estates.

Line 9: This line gives your Attorney(s)-in-Fact the right to handle claims and litigation for you, including to bring a lawsuit for you, to defend you against claims, and to settle disputes for you.

Line 10: This line gives your Attorney(s)-in-Fact authority to deal with your taxes. Although you might prefer to forget about this, it's important that tax forms be prepared and taxes paid, to avoid possible problems.

Line 11: This line authorizes your Attorney(s)-in-Fact to handle your personal affairs, to take steps to provide for the support and welfare of your family, and to maintain your relationships with family, friends, and organizations.

Line 12: This line enables your Attorney(s)-in-Fact to handle any matters you may have with the military, including making and receiving proceeds of any claims and maximizing benefits from military service.

Line 13: This line empowers your Attorney(s)-in-Fact to make, execute, file, store, and keep records, reports, and statements for you.

Line 14: This line allows your Attorney(s)-in-Fact to delegate his/her powers to someone else.

Line 15: This line is a general, catch-all authorizing your Attorney(s)-in-Fact to do anything you could do.

Paragraph 4: In the space that follows, you could add other provisions or limitations, but if you try to do this, you'd better make sure your additions or changes comply with the law.

Paragraph 5: If you have decided to name more than one Attorney-in-Fact, you should fill in the next blank either with the word "severally" or "jointly." "Severally" means that either of your Attorneys-in-Fact on his/her own will be able to exercise the powers provided in the Power of Attorney; "jointly" means that your Attorneys-in-Fact must act together to use your Power of Attorney.

Paragraph 6: The next section allows you to limit the duration of the Power of Attorney. Be careful—if you limit its duration and it expires, you might not be able to create a new one (if you've become incompetent).

Paragraph 7: You can and should nominate someone to act as a conservator of your estate in the event that a court decides a conservator is necessary. As explained in the Power of Attorney, a conservator is someone who will manage your financial affairs.

Finally, sign and date the document at the end before two witnesses and a notary. The notary fills in and signs the bottom portion. A notary is authorized by the state or federal government to administer oaths and attest to the authenticity of signatures.

STATUTORY SHORT FORM POWER OF ATTORNEY

NOTICE: THE POWERS GRANTED BY THIS DOCUMENT ARE BROAD AND SWEEPING. THEY ARE DEFINED IN SECTION 523.24. IF YOU HAVE ANY QUESTIONS ABOUT THESE POWERS, OBTAIN COMPETENT ADVICE. THE USE OF ANY OTHER OR DIFFERENT FORM OF POWER OF ATTORNEY DESIRED BY THE PARTIES IS ALSO PERMITTED. THIS POWER OF ATTORNEY MAY BE REVOKED BY YOU IF YOU LATER WISH TO DO SO. THIS POWER OF ATTORNEY AUTHORIZES BUT DOES NOT REQUIRE THE ATTORNEY-IN-FACT TO ACT FOR YOU.

Know All by These Presents, which are intended to constitute a STATUTORY SHORT FORM POWER ATTORNEY pursuant to Minnesota Statutes, section 523.23:

That I, _____,

(insert name and address of the principal)

do hereby appoint _____

_____,

(insert name and address of the attorney-in-fact or
each attorney-in-fact if more than one is designated)

my attorney(s)-in-fact to act (jointly):

(NOTE: If more than one attorney-in-fact is designated and the principal wishes each attorney-in-fact to be able to exercise the power conferred, delete the word "jointly." Failure to delete the word "jointly" will require the attorneys-in-fact to act unanimously.)

First: in my name, place and stead in any way which I myself could do, if I were personally present, with respect to the following matters as each of them is defined in section 523.24:

(To grant to the attorney-in-fact any of the following powers, make a check or "x" in the line in front of each power being granted. To delete any of the following powers, do not make a check or "x" in the line in front of the power. You may, but need not, cross out each power being deleted with a line drawn through it (or in similar fashion). Failure to make a check or "x" in the line in front of the power will have the effect of deleting the power unless the line in front of the power of (O) is checked or x-ed.)

Check or "x":

_____ (A)   real property transactions;

_____ (B)   tangible personal property transactions;

_____ (C)   bond, share and commodity transactions;

_____ (D)   banking transactions;

_____ (E)   business operating transactions;

_____ (F)   insurance transactions;

_____ (G)   beneficiary transactions;

_____ (H)   gift transactions;

_____ (I)   fiduciary transactions;

_____ (J)   claims and litigation;

_____ (K)   family maintenance;

_____ (L)   benefits from military service;

_____ (M)   records, reports, and statements;

_____ (N)   all other matters;

_____ (O)   all of the powers listed in (A) through (N) above.

Second: (You must indicate below whether or not this power of attorney will be effective if you become incompetent. Make a check or "x" in the line in front of the statement that expresses your intent.)

_____ This power of attorney shall continue to be effective if I become incompetent. It shall not be affected by my later disability or incompetency.

_____ This power of attorney shall not be effective if I become incompetent.

Third: (You must indicate below whether or not this power of attorney authorizes the attorney-in-fact to transfer your property directly to the attorney-in-fact. Make a check or "x" in the line in front of the statement that expresses your intent.)

_____ This power of attorney authorizes the attorney-in-fact to receive the transfer directly.

_____ This power of attorney does not authorize the attorney-in-fact to receive the transfer directly.

In Witness Whereof I have hereunto signed my name this _____ day of _____, 19___.

_____
(Signature of Principal)

Specimen Signature of Attorney(s)-in-Fact:

_____

Signed in the presence of: _____

_____
Witness

_____
Witness

CERTIFICATE OF NOTARY

STATE OF MINNESOTA   )
) SS:
COUNTY OF _____)

On the _____ day of _____, 19___, before me personally came _____, whose identity is well known to me to be the individual described in and who executed the foregoing instrument, and (he)(she) acknowledged to me that (he)(she) executed the same.

_____
Notary Public

My commission expires: _____

2

Statutory Short Form Power of Attorney
(Minnesota)

Instructions/Explanation

The explanations that follow should provide you with a clear understanding of the terms used in the Statutory Short Form Power of Attorney.

Notice: The notice confirms what the book has already stated: the powers given to your Attorney(s)-in-Fact are broad.

Introduction: On the first blank line, fill in your name and address (you are the "principal"—the person making the Power of Attorney).

On the next line(s), fill in the name(s) and address(es) of the person(s) to whom you are giving the Power of Attorney (called the "Agent(s)" or "Attorney(s)-in-Fact").

If you have decided to name more than one Attorney-in-Fact, you must decide whether to leave or to strike the word "jointly." If you want to require your Attorneys-in-Fact to act together to use the Power of Attorney, you should leave the word "jointly." But if you prefer to allow either of your Attorneys-in-Fact on his/her own to exercise the powers provided in the Power of Attorney, you must strike out the word "jointly."

The following lettered clauses specify broad powers providing your Attorney(s)-in-Fact with wide latitude to manage your affairs. Powers are separately enumerated to avoid any questions about whether you intended to authorize your Attorney(s)-in-Fact to undertake specific actions on your behalf. For any powers you wish to give to your Attorney(s)-in-Fact, you must place a check or "x" mark in the line before such power(s). Since you cannot foresee all the possible problems that could arise, you are usually better off giving your Attorney(s)-in-Fact the broadest possible powers.

Clause A: This clause gives your Attorney(s)-in-Fact broad authority to mortgage, sell, buy, accept, manage, lease, and/or otherwise deal with real estate, including your home.

Clause B: This clause permits your Attorney(s)-in-Fact broad authority to buy, sell, manage, receive, mortgage, lease, and/or otherwise handle transactions involving items of personal property.

Clause C: This clause lets your Attorney(s)-in-Fact invest in securities on your behalf and to manage, receive, sell, mortgage, and/or otherwise handle securities for you. This is broad enough to allow your Attorney(s)-in-Fact even to vote at stockholders meetings.

Clause D: This clause authorizes your Attorney(s)-in-Fact to handle banking transactions, including to open and manage accounts, CDs, and other instruments in financial institutions, to sign checks, to make withdrawals, and to have access to your safe-deposit box.

Clause E: This clause allows your Attorney(s)-in-Fact to engage in any business transactions for you.

Clause F: This clause authorizes your Attorney(s)-in-Fact to handle insurance matters for you, including obtaining, managing, maintaining, or terminating insurance, paying premiums, and obtaining benefits for you.

Clause G: This clause permits your Attorney(s)-in-Fact to act for you with respect to any matters in which you are or may be a beneficiary, including with respect to trusts, probate estates, guardianships, conservatorships, or escrows.

Clause H: This clause authorizes your Attorney(s)-in-Fact to make, complete, or otherwise handle any gift transactions for you.

Clause I: This clause allows your Attorney(s)-in-Fact to handle fiduciary matters for you, including estate administration, guardianship, and conservatorship activities.

Clause J: This clause gives your Attorney(s)-in-Fact the right to handle claims and litigation for you, including to bring a lawsuit for you, to defend you against claims, and to settle disputes for you.

Clause K: This clause authorizes your Attorney(s)-in-Fact to take steps to provide for the support and welfare of your family and to maintain your relationships with family, friends, and organizations.

Clause L: This clause enables your Attorney(s)-in-Fact to handle any matters you may have with the military, including making and receiving proceeds of any claims and maximizing benefits from military service.

Clause M: This clause empowers your Attorney(s)-in-Fact to make, execute, file, and store records, reports, and statements, including tax returns, for you.

Clause N: This clause is a general, catch-all authorizing your Attorney(s)-in-Fact to do anything you could do.

The next section is *crucial* to making your power of attorney *durable*, so that it remains valid at the time you will need it most—during your incapacity.

Check the first line, stating that the power of attorney *will* be effective if you become incompetent.

The last paragraph, beginning with the word "Third," allows you to choose whether or not your Attorney(s)-in-Fact will be permitted to transfer your property to himself/herself.

Finally, sign and date the document at the end before two witnesses and a notary. Have the Attorney(s)-in-Fact sign his or her name under yours. The notary fills in and signs the bottom portion. A notary is authorized by the state or federal government to administer oaths and attest to the authenticity of signatures.

STATUTORY SHORT FORM
DURABLE GENERAL POWER OF ATTORNEY

NOTICE: The powers granted by this document are broad and sweeping. They are defined in the Connecticut Statutory Short Form Power of Attorney Act, sections 1–42 to 1–56, inclusive, of the general statutes, which expressly permits the use of any other or different form of power of attorney desired by the parties concerned.

Know All Men by These Presents, which are intended to constitute a GENERAL POWER OF ATTORNEY pursuant to Connecticut Statutory Short Form Power of Attorney Act:

That I, _____,
(insert name and address of the principal)

do hereby appoint _____

_____

_____

_____,
(insert name and address of the agent, or
each agent, if more than one is designated)

my attorney(s)-in-fact TO ACT _____.

If more than one agent is designated and the principal wishes each agent alone to be able to exercise the power conferred, insert in this blank the word "severally." Failure to make any insertion or the insertion of the word "jointly" will require the agents to act jointly.

First: In my name, place and stead in any way which I myself could do, if I were personally present, with respect to the following matters as each of them is defined in the Connecticut Statutory Short Form Power of Attorney Act to the extent that I am permitted by law to act through an agent:

(Strike out and initial in the opposite box any one or more of the subdivisions as to which the principal does NOT desire to give the agent authority. Such elimination of any one or more of subdivisions (A) to (K), inclusive, shall automatically constitute an elimination also of subdivision (L).)

To strike out any subdivision the principal must draw a line through the text of that subdivision AND write his initials in the box opposite.

(A)	real estate transactions;	( )
(B)	chattel and goods transactions;	( )
(C)	bond, share and commodity transactions;	( )
(D)	banking transactions;	( )
(E)	business operating transactions;	( )
(F)	insurance transactions;	( )
(G)	estate transactions;	( )
(H)	claims and litigation;	( )
(I)	personal relationships and affairs;	( )
(J)	benefits from military service;	( )

(K)	records, reports and statements;	( )
(L)	all other matters;	( )

_____

_____

_____

(Special provisions and limitations may be included in the statutory short form power of attorney only if they conform to the requirements of the Connecticut Statutory Short Form Power of Attorney Act.)

Second: With full and unqualified authority to delegate any or all of the foregoing powers to any person or persons whom my attorney(s)-in-fact shall select;

Third: Hereby ratifying and confirming all that said attorney(s) or substitute(s) do or cause to be done.

This power of attorney shall not be affected by the subsequent disability or incompetence of the principal.

In Witness Whereof, I have hereunto signed my name and affixed my seal this _____ day of _____, 19___.

_____ (Seal)
(Signature of Principal)

Specimen Signature of Attorney(s)-in-Fact:

_____

Signed in the presence of:

_____

_____
Witness

_____
Witness

CERTIFICATE OF NOTARY

STATE OF CONNECTICUT   )
) SS:
COUNTY OF _____)

On the _____ day of _____, 19___, before me personally came _____, whose identity is well known to me to be the individual described in and who executed the foregoing instrument, and (he)(she) acknowledged to me that (he)(she) executed the same.

_____
Notary Public

My commission expires:

_____

Statutory Short Form
Durable General Power of Attorney
(Connecticut)

Instructions/Explanation

The explanations that follow should provide you with a clear understanding of the terms used in the Statutory Short Form Durable General Power of Attorney.

Notice: The notice confirms what the book has already stated: the powers given to your Attorney(s)-in-Fact are broad.

Introduction: On the first blank line, fill in your name and address (you are the "principal"—the person making the Durable General Power of Attorney).

On the next lines, fill in the name(s) and address(es) of the person(s) to whom you are giving the Durable General Power of Attorney (called the "Agent(s)" or "Attorney(s)-in-Fact").

If you have decided to name more than one Attorney-in-Fact, you should fill in the next blank either with the word "severally" or "jointly." "Severally" means that either of your Attorneys-in-Fact on his/her own will be able to exercise the powers provided in the Durable General Power of Attorney; "jointly" means that your Attorneys-in-Fact must act together to use your Durable General Power of Attorney.

The following lettered clauses specify broad powers providing your Attorney(s)-in-Fact with wide latitude to manage your affairs. Powers are separately enumerated to avoid any questions about whether you intended to authorize your Attorney(s)-in-Fact to undertake specific actions on your behalf. If you choose not to give all these powers to your Attorney(s)-in-Fact, you must draw a line through the power(s) that you want to exclude *and* initial inside the parentheses after such excluded power(s).

Clause A: This clause gives your Attorney(s)-in-Fact broad authority to mortgage, sell, buy, accept, manage, lease, and/or otherwise deal with real estate, including your home.

Clause B: This clause permits your Attorney(s)-in-Fact broad authority to buy, sell, manage, receive, mortgage, lease, and/or otherwise handle transactions involving items of personal property.

Clause C: This clause lets your Attorney(s)-in-Fact invest in securities on your behalf and manage, receive, sell, mortgage, and/or otherwise handle securities for you. This is broad enough to allow your Attorney(s)-in-Fact even to vote at stockholders meetings.

Clause D: This clause authorizes your Attorney(s)-in-Fact to handle banking transactions, including to open and manage accounts, CDs, and other instruments in financial institutions, to sign checks, to make withdrawals, and to have access to your safe-deposit box.

Clause E: This clause allows your Attorney(s)-in-Fact to engage in any business transactions for you.

Clause F: This clause authorizes your Attorney(s)-in-Fact to handle any insurance matters for you, including obtaining, managing, maintaining, or terminating insurance, paying premiums, and obtaining benefits for you.

Clause G: This clause permits your Attorney(s)-in-Fact to act for you with respect to estate matters, including receiving inheritances and participating in the administration of estates.

Clause H: This clause gives your Attorney(s)-in-Fact the right to handle claims and litigation for you, including to bring a lawsuit for you, to defend you against claims, and to settle disputes for you.

Clause I: This clause authorizes your Attorney(s)-in-Fact to handle your personal affairs, to take steps to provide for the support and welfare of your family, and to maintain your relationships with family, friends, and organizations.

Clause J: This clause enables your Attorney(s)-in-Fact to handle any matters you may have with the military, including making and receiving proceeds of any claims and maximizing benefits from military service.

Clause K: This clause empowers your Attorney(s)-in-Fact to make, execute, file, and store records, reports, and statements, including tax returns, for you.

Clause L: This clause is a general, catch-all authorizing your Attorney(s)-in-Fact to do anything you could do.

On the lines that follow, you could add other provisions or limitations, but if you try to do this, you'd better make sure your additions or changes comply with the law.

The paragraph beginning with "Second" allows your Attorney(s)-in-Fact to delegate his/her powers to someone else.

The paragraph beginning with "Third" provides that you ratify and confirm actions taken by your Attorney(s)-in-Fact under the Durable General Power of Attorney. This lets third parties know they can rely on your Attorney(s)-in-Fact's use of the document.

The next sentence is *crucial* to making your power of attorney *durable,* so that it remains valid at the time you will need it most—during your incapacity.

Finally, sign and date the document at the end before two witnesses and a notary. Have the Attorney(s)-in-Fact sign his or her name under yours. The notary fills in and signs the bottom portion. A notary is authorized by the state or federal government to administer oaths and attest to the authenticity of signatures.

Appendix B
Five Model Medicaid Trusts

Medicaid Trusts are as different as the people interested in setting them up. They can vary depending on the individual's particular circumstances and desires.

Following are five different model form Medicaid Trusts, each varying in important respects. You should examine them closely to see if any one fits your needs.

Following each Medicaid Trust form is an Instructions/Explanation sheet to clarify each provision in the trust agreement. To save flipping pages, much of the Instructions/Explanation is duplicated through the five forms.

IRREVOCABLE TRUST AGREEMENT

THIS IRREVOCABLE TRUST AGREEMENT is entered into at _____
_____, _____, this _____ day of _____, 19__, by and
between _____, of _____,
_____, the Settlor, hereinafter referred to in the first person,
and _____, of _____,
_____, the Trustee, hereinafter referred to as the "Trustee" and
sometimes in the third person impersonal.

ARTICLE I

CREATION OF TRUST

    A. Except as provided in Paragraph B of this Article I, this Trust Agreement shall be irrevocable, and I hereby expressly acknowledge that I shall have no right or power, either alone or in conjunction with others, and in any capacity whatsoever, to alter, amend, modify, revoke or terminate this Trust or any of the terms of this Trust Agreement in whole or in part, or otherwise to cause any of the assets of the Trust to revert to me or to my estate.

    B. I hereby transfer the property listed in Schedule A of this Trust Agreement to the Trustee. That property and all proceeds, investments and reinvestments thereof and any property hereinafter received by the Trustee from me, my **[wife/husband]**, _____, or from any other person (such property being hereinafter referred to as the "trust estate") shall be held, administered and distributed in accordance with the terms of the trust herein expressed. I reserve to myself and to others the right to add property to the trust estate by lifetime or testamentary gifts, all of which added property shall be governed by the terms hereof.

ARTICLE II

DISTRIBUTIONS DURING LIFETIME OF SETTLOR

    During my lifetime, the Trustee may distribute to or for the benefit of me or my **[wife/husband]**, _____, out of the net income of the trust estate, such amount or amounts as the Trustee deems necessary to provide for my and/or my said **[wife's/husband's]** maintenance and support. At the end of each taxable year the Trustee shall add any undistributed income to the principal of the trust estate being held hereunder.

ARTICLE III

DIVISION OF TRUST ESTATE UPON SETTLOR'S DEATH

    Upon my death, the Trustee shall hold, administer and distribute the property held hereunder, as the same shall be constituted after being (a) augmented by property received or to be received by the Trustee as a consequence of my death, including, without limitation, any property received or to be received under the terms of my Last Will and Testament or any Codicil thereto and (b) depleted by any money disbursed by the Trustee pursuant to the provisions of Paragraph C of Article VI hereof (said property as so constituted being hereinafter referred to as "The Family Trust") in accordance with the following provisions of this Trust Agreement.

A. Upon my death, if my **[wife/husband]**, _____, survives me:

    1. During my said **[wife's/husband's]** lifetime, the Trustee may distribute to or for the benefit of my said **[wife/husband]** such amount or amounts of the net income of The Family Trust as the Trustee deems necessary to provide for my said **[wife's/husband's]** maintenance and support. At the end of each taxable year, the Trustee shall add any undistributed income to the principal of the trust estate being held hereunder.

    2. Upon the death of my said **[wife/husband]**, the Trustee may pay to my said **[wife's/husband's]** estate cash and/or properties aggregating in value an amount or amounts requested in writing by the representative thereof, to pay and/or assist in satisfying my said **[wife's/husband's]** funeral expenses or the expenses of administration of **[her/his]** estate. The Trustee shall have no duty to ascertain or examine into the correctness of any amounts so requested, nor to see to the application of any funds paid over to **[her/his]** estate, the receipt of the representative thereof to be a complete acquittance to the Trustee hereunder with respect thereto. The balance of The Family Trust being held hereunder shall be distributed, subject to the provisions of Paragraph C of this Article III, in equal shares, to my then living children, treating as a then living child for this purpose the collective then living issue of any child of mine who shall then be deceased, the distribution to such issue to be *per stirpes*, the root of the *per stirpes* distribution to be such predeceased child.

B. Upon my death if my said **[wife/husband]** does not survive me, the Trustee, subject to the provisions of Paragraph C of this Article III, shall distribute the balance of The Family Trust being held hereunder, in equal shares, to my then living children, treating as a then living child the then living collective issue of any child of mine who shall then be deceased, the distribution to such issue to be *per stirpes*, the root of the *per stirpes* distribution to be such predeceased child.

C. If, under the provisions of Paragraphs A or B of this Article III, any portion of The Family Trust shall become distributable to any person who is then under the age of twenty-one (21) years, then such portion shall be retained by the Trustee in trust for the benefit of such person. The Trustee shall distribute to or for the benefit of such person out of the net income or principal or both of such portion held for such person, such amount or amounts (whether the whole or a lesser amount) as the Trustee, in its sole discretion, deems necessary or proper suitably to provide for the maintenance, support, health, and education of such person, and shall from time to time add to the principal of such portion the remaining undistributed income, if any, until such person shall attain the age of twenty-one (21) years, whereupon the Trustee shall distribute all of such portion to such person. If such person shall die prior to receiving the complete distribution of the portion held for such person's benefit, such portion shall be distributed free of the trust to such person's estate.

D. If at the time for distribution of The Family Trust or any share or portion of the trust estate being held pursuant to this Article III, there is no person or person's estate entitled under the provisions of this Article III other than this Paragraph D to take such distribution, the Trustee shall divide the trust estate into two (2) equal shares. One such share shall be distributed free of the trust to such person or persons as would be entitled to inherit from me and in the proportions they would so inherit under the laws of the State of _____ as though I had died intestate and domiciled in the State of _____ at the time distribution is so to be made. The other such share shall be distributed free of the trust to such person or persons as would be entitled to inherit from my said **[wife/husband]** and in the proportions they would so inherit under the laws of the State of _____ as though **[she/he]** had died intestate and domiciled in the State of _____ at the time distribution is so to be made.

E. If the Trustee is authorized pursuant to the provisions of this Article III to make distributions or payments to or for the benefit of any person (including distributions or payments directed or permitted to be made to a person who is under legal disability or, in the reasonable opinion of the Trustee, is unable properly to administer such distributions or payments), the Trustee may make such distributions or payments in any one or more of the following ways, as the Trustee may deem advisable: (1) directly to such beneficiary; (2) to the legal guardian of such beneficiary; (3) to any custodian then serving for such beneficiary, or to any person designated by the Trustee to serve as a custodian for such beneficiary (any such custodian may be the Trustee); or (4) by the Trustee itself expending such income or principal for the benefit of such beneficiary. The Trustee shall not be required to see to the application of any distribution or payment so made, but the receipt of any of the persons mentioned in Clause (1), (2) or (3) in the immediately preceding sentence shall be a full discharge for the Trustee.

F. All interests of a beneficiary hereunder shall be inalienable and free from anticipation, assignment, attachment, pledge or control by creditors or a present or former spouse of such beneficiary in any proceedings at law or in equity.

G. Any provisions of this Article III to the contrary notwithstanding, if not already distributed, all accrued and undistributed income and the entire principal of every trust estate then held hereunder shall be paid over and distributed outright and free of the trust not later than the end of the day immediately preceding the expiration of twenty-one (21) years from and after the death of the last survivor of myself, my said **[wife/husband]**, my children and my children's issue living at the time of the death of the first to die of my said **[wife/husband]** and me. Such payment and distribution shall be made to the person or persons for whose benefit the trust estate or estates respectively shall then be held hereunder.

ARTICLE IV

DETERMINATION OF SURVIVOR

If my **[wife/husband]**, _____, and I shall die under such circumstances that there is not sufficient evidence to determine the order of our deaths, or if **[she/he]** shall die within a period of thirty (30) days after the date of my death, then, for the purposes of this Trust Agreement, my said **[wife/husband]** shall be deemed not to have survived me.

ARTICLE V

DEFINITIONS

A. The words "issue," "child" and "children," as used herein, shall be deemed to include any legally adopted person as if he or she were the natural child of the adopting parent.

B. Whenever the context so requires, the use of words herein in the singular shall be construed to include the plural, and words in the plural, the singular, and words whether in the masculine, feminine or neuter gender shall be construed to include all of said genders.

ARTICLE VI

POWERS AND DUTIES OF THE TRUSTEE

A. There shall be no duty on the Trustee to pay or see to the payment of any premiums on any policies of life insurance or to take any steps to keep them in force, until such time as the Trustee holds title to any insurance policies hereunder as a part of the corpus of any trust estate. The Trustee furthermore assumes no responsibility with respect to the validity or enforceability of said policies. However, as soon as practicable after receiving notice of the death of the insured under any of such policies, the Trustee shall proceed to collect all amounts payable thereunder. The Trustee shall have full and complete authority to collect and receive any and all such amounts and its receipt therefor shall be a full and complete acquittance to any insurer or payor, who shall be under no obligation to see to the proper application thereof by the Trustee.

B. In the administration of the trusts created hereunder and in addition to the powers exercised by trustees generally, the Trustee shall have the following powers and authorities without any court order or proceeding, exercisable in the discretion of the Trustee:

1. To purchase as an investment for the trust estate or estates any property, real or personal, belonging to my estate and/or the estate of my **[wife/husband]**, _____;

2. To retain as suitable investments for the trust estate or estates any properties (including, without limitation, securities issued by any corporate Trustee or the holding company of which it is an affiliate) received by it from me, my said **[wife/ husband]**, my estate and/or the estate of my said **[wife/husband]**, and whether received by purchase or in any other manner, without regard to any law, statutory or judicial, or any rule or practice of court now or hereafter in force specifying or limiting the permissible investments of trustees, trust companies or fiduciaries generally or requiring the diversification of investments, and without liability to any person whomsoever for loss or depreciation in value thereof;

3. To sell, exchange, convey, mortgage, pledge, lease, control, and manage, and to make contracts concerning, any of the properties, real or personal, comprised in the trust estate or estates, all either publicly or privately and for such considerations and upon such terms as to credit or otherwise as may be reasonable under the circumstances, which leases and contracts may extend beyond the duration of any of the trusts created hereunder; to give options therefor; and to execute deeds, transfers, mortgages, leases and other instruments of any kind;

4. To invest and reinvest the properties from time to time comprised in the trust estate or estates in stocks, common and/or preferred, bonds, notes, debentures, loans, mortgages, common trust funds, or other securities or property, real or personal, all limitations now or hereafter imposed by law, statutory or judicial, or by any rule or practice of court now or hereafter in force specifying or limiting the permissible investments of trustees, trust companies or fiduciaries generally or requiring the diversification of investments, being hereby expressly waived, it being the intent hereof that the Trustee shall have full power and authority to deal with the trust estate or estates in all respects as though it was the sole owner thereof, without order of court or other authority;

5. To borrow money, from itself or otherwise, with or without security, whenever it deems such action advisable;

6. To exercise voting rights, execute and deliver powers of attorney and proxies and similarly act with reference to shares of stock and other securities comprised in the trust estate or estates in such manner as it deems proper, including, without limitation, the power to participate in or oppose reorganizations, recapitalizations, mergers, consolidations, exchanges, liquidations, arrangements and other corporate actions;

7. To collect all money; in accordance with generally accepted trust accounting principles, to determine whether money or other property coming into its possession shall be treated as principal or income and to charge or apportion expenses, taxes, gains and losses to principal or income;

8. To compromise, adjust and settle claims in favor of or against the trust estate or estates upon such terms and conditions as it may deem best; in the case of any litigation in connection with any part of such trust estate or estates, it may, under advice of its counsel, arbitrate, settle, or adjust any such matter in dispute upon such terms as it may consider just and equitable, and its decision shall be binding upon the beneficiaries;

9. To employ investment counsel, custodians of estate property, brokers, accountants, attorneys, clerical or bookkeeping assistants, and other suitable agents and to pay their reasonable compensation and expenses in addition to any compensation pay-

able to the Trustee, and to execute and deliver powers of attorney; the Trustee shall not be liable for any neglect, omission or wrongdoing of such investment counsel, custodians, brokers, accountants, attorneys, assistants or agents, provided reasonable care shall have been exercised in their selection;

10. To hold title to stocks, bonds, or other securities or property, real or personal, in its own name or in the name of its nominee and without indication of any fiduciary capacity or to hold any such bonds or securities in bearer form; the Trustee shall assume full responsibility for the acts of any nominee selected by it;

11. To make all repairs, alterations or improvements of any real property which shall constitute a part of the trust estate or estates; adjust boundaries thereof, and to erect or demolish buildings thereon; and, with respect to such property, to convert for different use, grant easements for adequate consideration, partition, and insure for any or all risks;

12. To pay premiums on any policies of life insurance which may form a part of the trust estate or estates; to cancel, sell, assign, hypothecate, pledge or otherwise dispose of any of said policies; to exercise any right, election, option or privilege granted by any of said policies; to borrow any sums in accordance with the provisions of any of said policies, and to receive all payments, dividends, surrender values, additions, benefits or privileges of any kind which may accrue to any of said policies;

13. To make any allocation, division or distribution required or permitted hereunder in cash or in kind, in real or personal property, or an undivided interest therein, or partly in cash and partly in kind, and to do so without making pro rata allocations, divisions or distributions of specific assets, property allocated, divided or distributed in kind to be taken at its fair market value at the time of such allocation, division or distribution;

14. To receive, in accordance with the provisions of Article I hereof, additional property from me or any other person, the Trustee being authorized and empowered to merge and hold as one any duplicate trusts held for the same beneficiary;

15. To make such expenditures and do such other acts as are reasonably required to manage, improve, protect, preserve, invest or sell any of the trust estates or otherwise properly to administer this Trust.

C. If the representative of my estate, in such representative's sole discretion, shall determine that appropriate assets of my estate are not available in sufficient amount to pay (a) taxes levied against or with respect to my taxable estate by reason of my death, including interest and penalties thereon, if any, and (b) expenses of administration of my estate, the Trustee shall, upon the request of the representative of my estate, contribute from the principal of the trust estate the amount of such deficiency; and in connection with any such action the Trustee shall rely upon the written statement of the representative of my estate as to the validity and correctness of the amounts of any such taxes, expenses and bequests, and shall furnish funds to such representative so as to enable such representative to discharge the same, or to discharge any part or all thereof themselves by making payment directly to the governmental official or agency or to the person entitled or claiming to be entitled to receive payment thereof. No consideration need be required by the Trustee from the representative of my estate for any disbursement made by the Trustee pursuant hereto, nor shall there be any obligation upon such representative to repay to the Trustee any of the funds disbursed by it hereunder, and all amounts disbursed by the Trustee pursuant to the authority hereby conferred upon it shall be disbursed without any right in or duty upon the Trustee to seek or obtain contribution or reimbursement from any person or property on account of such payment. The Trustee shall not be responsible for the application of any funds delivered by it to the representative of my estate pursuant to the authority herein granted, nor shall the Trustee be subject to liability to any beneficiary hereunder on account of any payment made by it pursuant to the provisions hereof.

D. The Trustee shall keep accurate records showing all receipts and disbursements and other transactions involving the trust estate or estates and shall furnish annually to each beneficiary currently entitled to income, (1) a statement of the receipts and disbursements affecting such beneficiary's interest in the trust, and (2) a complete inventory of the trust estate then held for the benefit of such beneficiary.

E. No person, firm or corporation dealing with the Trustee or a nominee of the Trustee or performing any act pursuant to action taken or order given by the Trustee or such nominee shall be obliged to inquire as to the propriety, validity or legality thereof hereunder, nor shall any such person be liable for the application of any money or other consideration paid to the Trustee or such nominee, but, instead, may rely upon any action taken by the Trustee or such nominee pursuant to the powers and authorities conferred upon it under the provisions of this Article VI in all respects as if the same were completely unlimited. No transfer agent or registrar of any security held hereunder shall be required to inquire as to the propriety, validity or legality of any transfer made by the Trustee or such nominee.

F. 1. In the event that said _____ shall be unwilling or unable to continue to serve as Trustee hereunder, then, my _____, _____, of _____, _____, shall serve as successor Trustee hereunder. In the event that both said _____ and said _____ shall be unwilling or unable to serve or continue to serve as Trustee hereunder, then _____, of _____, _____, shall serve as successor Trustee hereunder. Any Trustee shall be entitled to resign as Trustee for any reason whatsoever by giving written notice to the Trustee designated to succeed it; provided that the Trustee designated to succeed it shall first execute a formal written acceptance of the duties and obligations of the Trustee hereunder and file an executed copy of such acceptance with the preceding Trustee. After this is done, and when all sums then due from the trust estate to such predecessor Trustee have been paid, such predecessor Trustee shall transfer the Trust property then in its hands to such successor Trustee and such predecessor Trustee shall thereupon and thereby be discharged of all subsequent duties and obligations under or arising out of its trusteeship.

2. Any successor Trustee shall have and enjoy all the powers, authorities, duties and immunities hereby vested in and imposed upon the original Trustee and no successor Trustee shall be obliged to inquire into or be in any way accountable for the previous administration of the trust property.

G. My Trustee is authorized, in its discretion, to sell to, purchase from, borrow funds from, lend funds to, or otherwise deal with, upon such terms and conditions as my Trustee shall deem just and equitable and for full and adequate consideration, the Executor of the Last Will and Testament of myself or my said **[wife/husband]** or the Trustee of any Trust established by me or my said **[wife/husband]** (whether such Trust is a testamentary or inter vivos trust), even though my Trustee may also be serving as Executor under my Will or my said **[wife/husband]**'s Will or as Trustee under any such Trust established by me or by my said **[wife/husband]**.

H. In determining the amount of any discretionary distributions of income or principal to a beneficiary of a trust created hereunder, the Trustee shall be required to take into account all other means and resources known to or reasonably ascertainable by the Trustee, including Medicaid or any other form of government assistance, which are available to such beneficiary for the purposes for which the Trustee is authorized to make said distributions.

I. _____, as Trustee, shall serve without compensation. Any other Trustee shall be entitled to receive reasonable compensation. Any Trustee shall be entitled to be reimbursed for reasonable expenses it incurs which are necessary to carry out its duties as Trustee hereunder.

J. No bond shall be required of the Trustee hereunder or any successor Trustee.

K. The Trustee and any successor Trustee are specifically instructed by the Settlor to maintain the privacy and confidentiality of this instrument and the trust created hereunder, and are in no circumstances to divulge its terms to any probate or other court or other public agency with the exception of a tax authority.

L. The Trustee and any successor Trustee shall have the authority to merge any trust held hereunder with any other trust, however created, which has similar provisions, the same beneficiaries and the same Trustee.

M. Notwithstanding any other provision contained herein, an individual Trustee (a) shall have no incident of ownership or power with respect to any policy of insurance upon such Trustee's life, and (b) shall have no power of discretion with respect to the allocation or distribution of assets to the extent that such would discharge such Trustee's legal obligation to support any beneficiary, or directly or indirectly benefit such Trustee unless necessary to provide for such Trustee's support in reasonable comfort, health care or education at any level, considering such Trustee's other financial resources.

ARTICLE VII
GOVERNING LAW

This Trust Agreement shall be construed under and in accordance with the laws of the State of _____.

IN WITNESS WHEREOF, I have hereunto set my hand, and the Trustee, to evidence its acceptance of the Trust herein expressed, has hereunto set its hand, in duplicate, at _____, _____, _____, on the day and year first above written.

Signed in the presence of:

_____

_____   _____

                                                                      "Settlor"

_____   _____

_____   _____

                                                                      "Trustee"

I, the undersigned legal spouse of the Settlor, hereby waive all community property, dower or courtesy rights which I may have in the hereinabove-described property and give my assent to the provisions of the trust and to the inclusion in it of the said property.

_____

_____

Witness: _____   Witness: _____

STATE OF _____   City
                                            or
COUNTY OF _____   Town _____

On the _____ day of _____, 19____, personally appeared _____ known to me to be the individual(s) who executed the foregoing instrument, and acknowledged the same to be **[his/her]** free act and deed, before me.

My commission expires: _____   _____
                                                   Notary Public

7

SCHEDULE A

The following is a true and correct Schedule A of the property assigned, delivered and conveyed to _____, Trustee, to be held, treated and disposed of in accordance with the terms of a certain Irrevocable Trust Agreement between _____, the Settlor, and _____, the Trustee, dated _____ ____, 19___, to which Agreement this Schedule A is attached and made a part thereof.

_____

_____

_____

_____

_____

_____

_____

_____

_____

_____

_____

_____

_____

_____

_____

_____

Signed in the presence of:

_____   _____

_____   _____
                                                               "Settlor"

_____   _____

_____   _____
                                                               "Trustee"

    I, the undersigned legal spouse of the Settlor, hereby waive all community property, dower or courtesy rights which I may have in the hereinabove-described property and give my assent to the provisions of the trust and to the inclusion in it of the said property.

_____

_____

Witness: _____   Witness: _____

_____   _____

8

ADDITION OF PROPERTY TO IRREVOCABLE TRUST AGREEMENT
BY _____
DATED _____ ___, 19___
WITH _____, TRUSTEE
_____ (the "Assignor"), pursuant to the terms of the above-described Irrevocable Trust Agreement, does hereby assign, transfer and convey to ___, Trustee, and _____ _____, Trustee, does hereby acknowledge receipt of, the following assets from the Assignor:

_____
_____
_____
_____
_____
_____
_____
_____
_____
_____
_____
_____
_____
_____
_____
_____
_____
_____

The Trustee agrees to hold, manage and administer the above assets as a part of the trust estate created under such Irrevocable Trust Agreement.

At the request of the Trustee, the Assignor shall fully cooperate and execute any and all documents deemed necessary or desirable by it in order to cause the assignment made hereby to be properly recorded.

IN WITNESS WHEREOF, the Assignor and the Trustee have signed their names at _____, _____, on this ____ day of _____, 19___.

Signed in the presence of:

_____   _____

_____   _____, Assignor

_____   _____

_____   _____, Trustee

9

I, the undersigned legal spouse of the Assignor, hereby waive all community property, dower or courtesy rights which I may have in the hereinabove-described property and give my assent to the inclusion in the trust of the said property.

_____

_____

Witness: _____   Witness: _____

STATE OF _____   City
or
COUNTY OF _____   Town _____

On the _____ day of _____, 19___, personally appeared _____ known to me to be the individual(s) who executed the foregoing instrument, and acknowledged the same to be **[his/her]** free act and deed, before me.

_____
Notary Public

My commission expires:

_____

Medicaid Trust No. 1
for Individual Who Is Married, Distributing Assets to Children After Death of Both Spouses

Instructions/Explanation

As you can readily see, the trust agreement is filled with legalese. Don't be scared off by this confusing language. The explanations that follow should provide you with a clear understanding of the terms used.

Introduction: In the first blanks, fill in the city and state where you reside and the day, month, and year in which you are executing the Agreement.

Next, put in your name and residence (city and state)—the "Settlor" is your title when you make a trust. Then fill in the name, city, and state of the person or institution whom you are naming as trustee.

Remember, neither you nor your spouse should be the trustee. A child or other close relative will probably be your first choice (keeping in mind possible tax consequences where annual distributions of over $10,000 will be made). If no one fits that description, you may have to name an institutional trustee, such as a bank.

Article I(A): This is the section making your trust irrevocable. Once you sign the Agreement, you will never be able to change, amend, or revoke it.

Article I(B): This paragraph transfers into the Trust all the items listed on Schedule A at the end of the Agreement. You can include on Schedule A just about any item imaginable, including real estate, personal property, savings and checking accounts, boats, cars, even clothing.

If the property you put into the trust increases in value, the increased value is part of the trust. And if an asset changes form, the new asset still remains in the trust. For example, if the trustee takes $5,000 from a bank account and buys $5,000 worth of stock, the stock remains in the trust.

While you can never remove assets once they are placed into the trust, you can always add to the trust by using the Addition to Trust form following Schedule A.

A testamentary gift, referred to in this paragraph, is a gift given at the time of someone's death, normally contained in a will. For example, you may not put your car into trust immediately, but you may add to your trust under your will when you die.

IMPORTANT NOTE: In Paragraph I(B) and throughout this Trust Agreement, you will see references to [wife/husband]. If your spouse is a female, strike out husband; if a male, strike out wife. On the line following [wife/husband], fill in the name.

Article II: This section gives you and your spouse the income from the trust during your lives, but specifically provides that you cannot get at the principal. This is *absolutely crucial* to saving your estate from the grasp of a nursing home if either you or your spouse enters one. With this language, Medicaid cannot require you to spend the principal on the nursing home *because you don't control or even have access to the principal*.

Why does the Trust Agreement give discretion to the Trustee to pay you and/or your spouse income rather than requiring the Trustee to pay all the income? Because with this provision, you *may* be able to protect your income from the nursing home.

Let's say the Trust Agreement just said that all the income was automatically yours. If you entered a nursing home, Medicaid would force you to pay all the income to the nursing home and would only cover any deficiency on the bill. But if the Trustee has discretion to pay all the income to you or your spouse, after you go into a nursing home the Trustee might decide to pay all the income to your spouse and none to you. In that situation, Medicaid might pay the entire nursing-home tab, because you don't have any income. (I say might because the law and its application to situations like this are not yet clear. It is possible that Medicaid might say that, even if you're not actually receiving any income, you *could* receive some or all of the income and so it won't pay the full nursing-home bill.)

Article III: This section describes how your trust principal, less any of your estate taxes, estate administration costs, or funeral expenses as provided in

Article VI(C), will be distributed after you and/or your spouse die.

Paragraph III(A)(1) provides that, if you die before your spouse, your spouse gets the income from the trust during his/her lifetime. Your spouse can't get at the principal during her life, so that if he/she goes into a nursing home, the principal will remain protected for your heirs.

Then when your spouse dies, Paragraph III(A)(2) says that the balance of your trust principal will be distributed equally to your children who are living at the time of your spouse's death. If any of your children has died before your spouse passed away, that child's portion goes to that child's children.

Paragraph III(B) provides for the distribution of the trust principal if you die after your spouse. The distribution is the same as under III(A)(2), to your children in equal shares.

Paragraph III(C) provides that, if any person who is to receive a distribution is under age twenty-one, that person's distribution shall be kept in trust until that person reaches age twenty-one. This provision allows you to make sure that, if you have a young child or grandchild who is to receive a distribution from your trust, that child cannot have control of the funds until he/she is old enough (and, it is hoped, mature enough) to manage those funds. This trust provides for distribution of a child's portion upon reaching age twenty-one, although any age could be chosen and inserted into the trust.

Paragraph III(D) provides for the distribution of the trust if there's no one to receive the principal from your trust under Paragraphs III(A) or (B). If you and your spouse die leaving no living children or grandchildren, Paragraph III(D) takes over.

Under III(D), the remaining principal of the trust will be divided into two parts. One part will go to those persons who would inherit from you under the laws of your state as if you had died without a will or a trust. Every state has a law that dictates to whom an estate of someone who dies without a will will be distributed—usually to the closest living relative(s) of the deceased. For example, if you die without children or grandchildren, Paragraph III(D) may mean that your parent or brother collects part of the trust estate.

The other half of the trust estate will be distributed to those persons who would inherit from your deceased spouse under the laws of your state as if he or she had died without a will.

The estate is split into two parts so that relatives on both sides of your family are treated equally. For example, rather than having everything go to your cousin, half may go to your cousin and half to your deceased spouse's sister.

Fill in the blanks in Paragraph III(D) with the name of your state.

Part III(E) discusses distributions, after you die, to beneficiaries named in your trust who are under some legal disability or are unable to administer their distributions. For example, if your spouse is senile or suffering from Alzheimer's disease, he or she may be under a legal disability or unable to manage his or her money.

If a distribution from your trust is to go to someone who is under a legal disability or unable to manage their money, the Trustee has four options:

1. Pay the money to the beneficiary.
2. Make the distribution to a legal guardian of the beneficiary.
3. Distribute the beneficiary's portion to a custodian for the beneficiary.
4. Spend the money himself or herself for the benefit of the beneficiary.

If, when you make up your trust, you could predict the ages and physical and mental conditions of all your beneficiaries at the time of your death, you could spell out which of these four options you would want the Trustee to pursue. But since you can't, this Trust allows the Trustee to choose which option he or she believes is best.

The last sentence of Part III(E) says that, once the Trustee has made his or her choice and distributed a beneficiary's portion to the beneficiary or to the beneficiary's guardian or custodian, the Trustee is off the hook; he or she doesn't have to monitor the use of the distribution after that.

Part III(F), often called a spendthrift clause, provides that nobody but your intended beneficiary can obtain an interest in a distribution under your Trust. For example, your child, who will receive a portion of your Trust after you're gone, can't sell his or her expected distribution in the future to someone for cash now. And a beneficiary can't put up his or her interest in a distribution as collateral for a loan. After all, you want the person you name in the Trust to receive a distribution, not some stranger.

Spendthrift clauses like this are enforced in most, but not all, states. If you have a serious concern that a beneficiary has or may have creditor problems, consult with a local attorney to determine whether this clause will be effective in your state.

Trusts cannot legally tie up assets forever, so Part III(G) is designed to avoid potential problems by limiting the life of the Trust.

Article IV: Let's say you and your spouse are killed in an accident together. One of you must have died minutes before the other. Rather than leave open the possibility of confusion over who died first, this paragraph says that your spouse will be considered to have died first.

Article V: This is the definition section. The only important point here is to recognize that a legally adopted child will be considered a child for purposes of the Trust Agreement. So by leaving everything to your children equally after you and your spouse die, any adopted child would be treated the same as a natural child.

Article VI: This section deals with the powers and duties you are giving to the Trustee.

Part VI(A) says that, after your death, the Trustee must collect the money due under any insurance policy on your life. The Trustee does not have a duty to pay your life insurance premiums during your lifetime, until and unless the Trustee takes title to any insurance policy.

Part VI(B) is very important, setting forth the powers of the Trustee. As you can see, this Trust Agreement gives the Trustee very broad powers to administer the funds and property in the estate, including the power to:

1. Buy real estate or personal property from your or your spouse's estate. Without this power, purchases by your Trustee from your estate at death might not be allowed.
2. Keep in the Trust anything received from you, your spouse, or your and your spouse's estates.
3. Sell, exchange, mortgage, and do just about anything else with property in the Trust.
4. Invest the assets in the Trust in just about anything.
5. Borrow money for the Trust.
6. Manage stock and other securities.
7. Collect money for the Trust.
8. Handle claims and lawsuits for or against the Trust.
9. Hire and pay counselors and assistants, like lawyers and accountants, for the Trust.
10. Hold property in his or her own name, in the name of a nominee, or in bearer form.
11. Manage real estate in the Trust, including repairing, improving, or converting property.
12. Handle life insurance policies in the Trust, including paying premiums, cancelling or selling policies, cashing in policies, or borrowing against them.
13. Make distributions under the Trust in cash or in property.
14. Receive additional property for the Trust.
15. Do anything else reasonably required to manage, protect, or preserve the Trust assets.

Why put in many specific powers, instead of just having item 15, which generally allows the Trustee to do anything reasonably necessary? Because with only a general statement, someone with whom the Trustee must deal may question his or her power and may refuse to do business with him or her. For example, without specifically giving the Trustee the power to sell real estate, buyers, lenders, and escrow agents may be hesitant to deal with him or her, even if your trust agreement generally gives him or her broad powers. By listing specific powers, you can ensure the Trustee's ability properly to manage the Trust.

Why give the Trustee such broad powers anyway? Why not just specify a few actions he or she may take? The reason is simple: you can't predict what the Trustee may need to do to manage your estate properly, and if you don't give him or her broad powers, you may hamper him or her and damage your Trust estate. For example, if you don't own any stocks, why give the Trustee power to manage them? Because at some point it might be in your best interest for your Trustee to purchase securities and your Trust Agreement could unnecessarily prevent him or her from doing so.

Part VI(C) provides for certain payments from your Trust upon your death. If the representative of your estate (such as the executor or administrator) decides that the funds left in your estate (not in your Trust) are insufficient to pay your estate taxes, expenses of administration, or funeral expenses, he or she can require the Trustee to cover those costs. The Trustee does not have to get anything in return, and your estate representative does not have to repay the money. Once the Trustee has paid the representative of your estate, the Trustee has no further obligation to monitor the use of these funds.

Part VI(D) requires the Trustee to keep accurate records showing all transactions in the Trust. Every year, the Trustee must give to certain beneficiaries a statement listing the Trust transactions for the year and a current inventory of assets in the Trust. Not every possible future beneficiary of the Trust gets this report. For example, if the Trust Agreement provides income to you for your lifetime, then on your death the assets will be distributed to your children or their children, only you are entitled to the Trustee's report.

Part VI(E) is designed to encourage people to deal with the Trustee by relieving them of liability in case the Trustee takes some action beyond his power. For example, if the Trustee attempts to sell a house, the buyer can go ahead with the transaction and pay the Trustee without worrying about whether the Trust really allows the Trustee to make that deal.

Part VI(F)(1) allows you to name alternative Trustees in case your first and/or second choice can't or won't serve when the time comes. In the first blank, put the name of your first choice for Trustee. In the next three blanks, fill in the relationship to you, the name and residence of your second choice. In the next two blanks, fill in the names of your first and second choices for Trustee. In the last three blanks, include the name, city, and state of a third choice for Trustee.

Part VI(F)(2) gives any successor Trustee all the same powers and duties as the original Trustee. It also encourages your chosen successor Trustee to accept the job by providing that he or she has no responsibility for anything done by the earlier Trustee.

Part VI(G) authorizes the Trustee to engage in transactions with the Executor of your or your spouse's estate or any trustee of any other trust established by you or your spouse. Without this language, a conflict-of-interest issue could arise over these types of dealings.

Part VI(H) concerns discretionary distributions by the Trustee. Under Article II, the Trustee is given discretion to distribute to you and your spouse all the net income of the trust. Let's say one of you enters a nursing home—will some or all of the income from the trust have to be paid to the nursing home? Under the law as it stands now, the answer is not totally clear. Medicaid may take the position that at least half and maybe *all* of the income must

be paid to the nursing-home spouse (and so to the nursing home). But with Part VI(H), there is a chance you can save part or all of the income.

Under Part VI(H), the Trustee could decide to pay all the income to the spouse-at-home. In fact, by requiring the Trustee to consider other resources available, including Medicaid, you are tilting the Trustee's decision in the direction of your spouse. If the Trustee makes that decision, Medicaid might allow the outside spouse to retain the income while it pays the institutional spouse's costs.

In Part VI(I), you are providing that the Trustee (whose name must be filled in the blank) will serve without compensation. Since the Trustee will probably be your child or someone else close to you, that should be agreeable. Other possible trustees, such as a bank, will want to be paid, and Part VI(I) allows that as well.

Part VI(J) states that the Trustee does not have to post a bond. A bond is like an insurance policy, designed to protect your Trust in case the Trustee does something wrong, such as steals assets. Depending on the amount in the Trust, the bond could easily cost your Trust several hundred dollars. If you've followed the tips in this book and selected the right Trustee, you shouldn't need a bond.

Part VI(K) instructs the Trustee to keep the terms of your Trust private to the maximum extent possible. A trust has a great advantage over a will when it comes to passing your assets along after your death. Your estate becomes an open book when it goes through probate; when it passes under a trust, it can be kept from the eyes of nosy neighbors.

Part VI(L) allows the Trustee to merge trusts that are very similar to avoid duplication of effort and costs.

Part VI(M) is a protection for the Trustee to avoid the remote possibility of having the trust property included in the Trustee's estate, causing adverse tax consequences.

Article VII: Article VII states that any questions about the Trust will be answered by the laws of the state of your primary residence. In the blank space, fill in the name of your state.

Conclusion: In the blanks in the final paragraph, fill in your city and state. Then sign where it says Settlor (that's you) and have the Trustee sign below that. You and the Trustee should each print your names below the signature lines. To the left of your and the Trustee's signatures, two witnesses to each signature must sign. The witnesses can be the same, but they don't have to be; if they are the same, they must sign twice (once for the Settlor and once for the Trustee). The witnesses cannot be members of your family.

Then your spouse should also sign, and two witnesses must sign below. In many states, your spouse has a legal interest in your property and must waive his or her rights in writing to the property covered by the trust.

The final section is for a notary public.

Schedule A: Following the end of the Trust is Schedule A, on which you should list any items (i.e., cash accounts, real estate, personal property, etc.) to be placed under the control of the Trustee. Identify each item as best you can, using addresses, registration numbers, account numbers, etc., wherever possible, to avoid confusion.

On Schedule A, fill in: the name of the Trustee in the first blank, your name (the "Settlor") in the second blank, and the name of the Trustee again in the third blank. Then date the Schedule.

At the bottom, you, the Trustee, and your spouse should sign before two independent witnesses.

Addition of Property Form: Finally included is a form that you can use to add property to the Trust later. At the top, fill in your name, the date that the Trust was originally made, and the name of the Trustee. In the first full paragraph, fill in your name as the Assignor, assigning property to the Trustee. Then on the lines that follow, list any items to be added to the Trust. Again, identify each item as best you can. At the end, you, the Trustee, and your spouse should sign before two independent witnesses and a notary.

IRREVOCABLE TRUST AGREEMENT

THIS IRREVOCABLE TRUST AGREEMENT is entered into at _____ _____, _____, this _____ day of _____, 19__, by and between _____, of _____, _____, the Settlor, hereinafter referred to in the first person, and _____, of _____, _____, the Trustee, hereinafter referred to as the "Trustee" and sometimes in the third person impersonal.

ARTICLE I

CREATION OF TRUST

A. Except as provided in Paragraph B of this Article I, this Trust Agreement shall be irrevocable, and I hereby expressly acknowledge that I shall have no right or power, either alone or in conjunction with others, and in any capacity whatsoever, to alter, amend, modify, revoke or terminate this Trust or any of the terms of this Trust Agreement in whole or in part, or otherwise to cause any of the assets of the Trust to revert to me or to my estate.

B. I hereby transfer the property listed in Schedule A of this Trust Agreement to the Trustee. That property and all proceeds, investments and reinvestments thereof and any property hereinafter received by the Trustee from me, my **[wife/husband]**, _____, or from any other person (such property being hereinafter referred to as the "trust estate") shall be held, administered and distributed in accordance with the terms of the trust herein expressed. I reserve to myself and to others the right to add property to the trust estate by lifetime or testamentary gifts, all of which added property shall be governed by the terms hereof.

ARTICLE II

DISTRIBUTIONS DURING LIFETIME OF SETTLOR

During my lifetime, the Trustee may distribute to or for the benefit of me or my **[wife/husband]**, _____, out of the net income of the trust estate, such amount or amounts as the Trustee deems necessary to provide for my and/or my said **[wife's/husband's]** maintenance and support. At the end of each taxable year the Trustee shall add any undistributed income to the principal of the trust estate being held hereunder.

ARTICLE III

DIVISION OF TRUST ESTATE UPON SETTLOR'S DEATH

Upon my death, the Trustee shall hold, administer and distribute the property held hereunder, as the same shall be constituted after being (a) augmented by property received or to be received by the Trustee as a consequence of my death, including, without limitation, any property received or to be received under the terms of my Last Will and Testament or any Codicil thereto and (b) depleted by any money disbursed by the Trustee pursuant to the provisions of Paragraph C of Article VI hereof (said property as so constituted being hereinafter referred to as "The Family Trust") in accordance with the following provisions of this Trust Agreement.

1

A. Upon my death, if my **[wife/husband]**, _____,
survives me:

1. During my said **[wife's/husband's]** lifetime, the Trustee may distribute to or for the benefit of my said **[wife/husband]** such amount or amounts of the net income of The Family Trust as the Trustee deems necessary to provide for my said **[wife's/husband's]** maintenance and support. At the end of each taxable year, the Trustee shall add any undistributed income to the principal of the trust estate being held hereunder.

2. Upon the death of my said **[wife/husband]**, the Trustee may pay to my said **[wife's/husband's]** estate cash and/or properties aggregating in value an amount or amounts requested in writing by the representative thereof, to pay and/or assist in satisfying my said **[wife's/husband's]** funeral expenses or the expenses of administration of **[her/his]** estate. The Trustee shall have no duty to ascertain or examine into the correctness of any amounts so requested, nor to see to the application of any funds paid over to **[her/his]** estate, the receipt of the representative thereof to be a complete acquittance to the Trustee hereunder with respect thereto. The balance of The Family Trust being held hereunder shall be held, administered and distributed pursuant to the provisions of Paragraph B of this Article III.

B. Upon the death of my said **[wife/husband]** if **[she/he]** survives me, or upon my death if my said **[wife/husband]** does not survive me, the Trustee shall divide the balance of The Family Trust being held hereunder into equal separate shares, one such share to be for the benefit of each then living child of mine, treating as a then living child of mine for this purpose the then living collective issue *per stirpes* of any child of mine who shall then be deceased, the root of the *per stirpes* division to be such deceased child. Said shares provided for in this Paragraph B shall be held, administered and distributed as follows:

1. The Trustee shall distribute forthwith any share created for the benefit of the then living collective issue of any child of mine who shall be deceased at the time of such division, to such issue *per stirpes*, the root of the *per stirpes* distribution to be such deceased child.

2. During the lifetime of any child of mine who survives my said **[wife/husband]** and me, the Trustee shall distribute to or for the benefit of such child, out of the net income or principal or both of the share held for the benefit of such child, such amount or amounts (whether the whole or a lesser amount) as the Trustee, in its sole discretion, deems necessary or proper suitably to provide for such child's maintenance, support, health, and education. Any undistributed income shall from time to time be added to the principal of the share held for the benefit of such child.

3. If any child of mine shall die prior to the complete distribution of the separate share held for the benefit of such child, such separate share shall be distributed to the following:
   (a) Such child's then living collective issue, to such issue *per stirpes*, the root of the *per stirpes* distribution to be such deceased child; or if there be no such issue then living, then to
   (b) The then living collective issue of such child's nearest ancestor (including myself as such an ancestor) of whom issue are then living provided such issue are issue of mine, to such issue *per stirpes*, the root of the *per stirpes* distribution to be such ancestor.

C. If at the time for distribution of The Family Trust or any share or portion of the trust estate being held pursuant to this Article III, there is no person or person's estate entitled under the provisions of this Article III other than this Paragraph C to take such distribution, the Trustee shall divide the trust estate into two (2) equal shares. One such share shall be distributed free of the trust to such person or persons as would be entitled to inherit from me and in the proportions they would so inherit under the laws of the State of _____ as though I had died intestate and domiciled in the State of _____ at the time distribution is so to be made. The other such share shall be distributed free of the trust to such person or persons as would be entitled to inherit from my said **[wife/husband]** and in the proportions they would so inherit under the laws of the State of _____ _____ as though **[she/he]** had died intestate and domiciled in the State of _____ at the time distribution is so to be made.

D. If the Trustee is authorized pursuant to the provisions of this Article III to make distributions or payments to or for the benefit of any person (including distributions or payments directed or permitted to be made to a person who is under legal disability or, in the reasonable opinion of the Trustee, is unable properly to administer such distributions or payments), the Trustee may make such distributions or payments in any one or more of the following ways, as the Trustee may deem advisable: (1) directly to such beneficiary; (2) to the legal guardian of such beneficiary; (3) to any custodian then serving for such beneficiary, or to any person designated by the Trustee to serve as a custodian for such beneficiary (any such custodian may be the Trustee); or (4) by the Trustee itself expending such income or principal for the benefit of such beneficiary. The Trustee shall not be required to see to the application of any distribution or payment so made, but the receipt of any of the persons mentioned in Clause (1), (2) or (3) in the immediately preceding sentence shall be a full discharge for the Trustee.

E. All interests of a beneficiary hereunder shall be inalienable and free from anticipation, assignment, attachment, pledge or control by creditors or a present or former spouse of such beneficiary in any proceedings at law or in equity.

F. Any provisions of this Article III to the contrary notwithstanding, if not already distributed, all accrued and undistributed income and the entire principal of every trust estate then held hereunder shall be paid over and distributed outright and free of the trust not later than the end of the day immediately preceding the expiration of twenty-one (21) years from and after the death of the last survivor of myself, my said **[wife/husband]**, my children and my children's issue living at the time of the death of the first to die of my said **[wife/husband]** and me. Such payment and distribution shall be made to the person or persons for whose benefit the trust estate or estates respectively shall then be held hereunder.

ARTICLE IV

DETERMINATION OF SURVIVOR

If my **[wife/husband]**, _____, and I shall die under such circumstances that there is not sufficient evidence to determine the order of our deaths, or if **[she/he]** shall die within a period of thirty (30) days after the date of my death, then, for the purposes of this Trust Agreement, my said **[wife/husband]** shall be deemed not to have survived me.

ARTICLE V

DEFINITIONS

A. The words "issue," "child" and "children," as used herein, shall be deemed to include any legally adopted person as if he or she were the natural child of the adopting parent.

B. Whenever the context so requires, the use of words herein in the singular shall be construed to include the plural, and words in the plural, the singular, and words whether in the masculine, feminine or neuter gender shall be construed to include all of said genders.

ARTICLE VI

POWERS AND DUTIES OF THE TRUSTEE

A. There shall be no duty on the Trustee to pay or see to the payment of any premiums on any policies of life insurance or to take any steps to keep them in force, until such time as the

3

Trustee holds title to any insurance policies hereunder as a part of the corpus of any trust estate. The Trustee furthermore assumes no responsibility with respect to the validity or enforceability of said policies. However, as soon as practicable after receiving notice of the death of the insured under any of such policies, the Trustee shall proceed to collect all amounts payable thereunder. The Trustee shall have full and complete authority to collect and receive any and all such amounts and its receipt therefor shall be a full and complete acquittance to any insurer or payor, who shall be under no obligation to see to the proper application thereof by the Trustee.

B. In the administration of the trusts created hereunder and in addition to the powers exercised by trustees generally, the Trustee shall have the following powers and authorities without any court order or proceeding, exercisable in the discretion of the Trustee:

1. To purchase as an investment for the trust estate or estates any property, real or personal, belonging to my estate and/or the estate of my **[wife/husband]**, _____;

2. To retain as suitable investments for the trust estate or estates any properties (including, without limitation, securities issued by any corporate Trustee or the holding company of which it is an affiliate) received by it from me, my said **[wife/husband]**, my estate and/or the estate of my said **[wife/husband]**, and whether received by purchase or in any other manner, without regard to any law, statutory or judicial, or any rule or practice of court now or hereafter in force specifying or limiting the permissible investments of trustees, trust companies or fiduciaries generally or requiring the diversification of investments, and without liability to any person whomsoever for loss or depreciation in value thereof;

3. To sell, exchange, convey, mortgage, pledge, lease, control, and manage, and to make contracts concerning, any of the properties, real or personal, comprised in the trust estate or estates, all either publicly or privately and for such considerations and upon such terms as to credit or otherwise as may be reasonable under the circumstances, which leases and contracts may extend beyond the duration of any of the trusts created hereunder; to give options therefor; and to execute deeds, transfers, mortgages, leases and other instruments of any kind;

4. To invest and reinvest the properties from time to time comprised in the trust estate or estates in stocks, common and/or preferred, bonds, notes, debentures, loans, mortgages, common trust funds, or other securities or property, real or personal, all limitations now or hereafter imposed by law, statutory or judicial, or by any rule or practice of court now or hereafter in force specifying or limiting the permissible investments of trustees, trust companies or fiduciaries generally or requiring the diversification of investments, being hereby expressly waived, it being the intent hereof that the Trustee shall have full power and authority to deal with the trust estate or estates in all respects as though it was the sole owner thereof, without order of court or other authority;

5. To borrow money, from itself or otherwise, with or without security, whenever it deems such action advisable;

6. To exercise voting rights, execute and deliver powers of attorney and proxies and similarly act with reference to shares of stock and other securities comprised in the trust estate or estates in such manner as it deems proper, including, without limitation, the power to participate in or oppose reorganizations, recapitalizations, mergers, consolidations, exchanges, liquidations, arrangements and other corporate actions;

7. To collect all money; in accordance with generally accepted trust accounting principles, to determine whether money or other property coming into its possession shall be treated as principal or income and to charge or apportion expenses, taxes, gains and losses to principal or income;

8. To compromise, adjust and settle claims in favor of or against the trust estate or

estates upon such terms and conditions as it may deem best; in the case of any litigation in connection with any part of such trust estate or estates, it may, under advice of its counsel, arbitrate, settle, or adjust any such matter in dispute upon such terms as it may consider just and equitable, and its decision shall be binding upon the beneficiaries;

9. To employ investment counsel, custodians of estate property, brokers, accountants, attorneys, clerical or bookkeeping assistants, and other suitable agents and to pay their reasonable compensation and expenses in addition to any compensation payable to the Trustee, and to execute and deliver powers of attorney; the Trustee shall not be liable for any neglect, omission or wrongdoing of such investment counsel, custodians, brokers, accountants, attorneys, assistants or agents, provided reasonable care shall have been exercised in their selection;

10. To hold title to stocks, bonds, or other securities or property, real or personal, in its own name or in the name of its nominee and without indication of any fiduciary capacity or to hold any such bonds or securities in bearer form; the Trustee shall assume full responsibility for the acts of any nominee selected by it;

11. To make all repairs, alterations or improvements of any real property which shall constitute a part of the trust estate or estates; adjust boundaries thereof, and to erect or demolish buildings thereon; and, with respect to such property, to convert for different use, grant easements for adequate consideration, partition, and insure for any or all risks;

12. To pay premiums on any policies of life insurance which may form a part of the trust estate or estates; to cancel, sell, assign, hypothecate, pledge or otherwise dispose of any of said policies; to exercise any right, election, option or privilege granted by any of said policies; to borrow any sums in accordance with the provisions of any of said policies, and to receive all payments, dividends, surrender values, additions, benefits or privileges of any kind which may accrue to any of said policies;

13. To make any allocation, division or distribution required or permitted hereunder in cash or in kind, in real or personal property, or an undivided interest therein, or partly in cash and partly in kind, and to do so without making pro rata allocations, divisions or distributions of specific assets, property allocated, divided or distributed in kind to be taken at its fair market value at the time of such allocation, division or distribution;

14. To receive, in accordance with the provisions of Article I hereof, additional property from me or any other person, the Trustee being authorized and empowered to merge and hold as one any duplicate trusts held for the same beneficiary;

15. To make such expenditures and do such other acts as are reasonably required to manage, improve, protect, preserve, invest or sell any of the trust estates or otherwise properly to administer this Trust.

C. If the representative of my estate, in such representative's sole discretion, shall determine that appropriate assets of my estate are not available in sufficient amount to pay (a) taxes levied against or with respect to my taxable estate by reason of my death, including interest and penalties thereon, if any, and (b) expenses of administration of my estate, the Trustee shall, upon the request of the representative of my estate, contribute from the principal of the trust estate the amount of such deficiency; and in connection with any such action the Trustee shall rely upon the written statement of the representative of my estate as to the validity and correctness of the amounts of any such taxes, expenses and bequests, and shall furnish funds to such representative so as to enable such representative to discharge the same, or to discharge any part or all thereof themselves by making payment directly to the governmental official or agency or to the person entitled or claiming to be entitled to receive payment thereof. No consideration need be required by the Trustee from the representative of my estate for any disbursement made by the Trustee pursuant hereto, nor shall there be any obligation upon such representative to repay to the Trustee any of the funds disbursed by it hereunder, and all amounts disbursed by the Trustee pursuant to the authority hereby conferred upon it shall be disbursed without any right in or duty upon the Trustee to seek or obtain contribution or reimbursement from any person or property on account of such payment. The Trustee shall not be responsible for the application of any funds delivered by it to the representative of my estate pursuant to the authority herein granted, nor shall the Trustee be subject to liability to any beneficiary hereunder on account of any payment made by it pursuant to the provisions hereof.

D. The Trustee shall keep accurate records showing all receipts and disbursements and other transactions involving the trust estate or estates and shall furnish annually to each beneficiary currently entitled to income, (1) a statement of the receipts and disbursements affecting such beneficiary's interest in the trust, and (2) a complete inventory of the trust estate then held for the benefit of such beneficiary.

E. No person, firm or corporation dealing with the Trustee or a nominee of the Trustee or performing any act pursuant to action taken or order given by the Trustee or such nominee shall be obliged to inquire as to the propriety, validity or legality thereof hereunder, nor shall any such person be liable for the application of any money or other consideration paid to the Trustee or such nominee, but, instead, may rely upon any action taken by the Trustee or such nominee pursuant to the powers and authorities conferred upon it under the provisions of this Article VI in all respects as if the same were completely unlimited. No transfer agent or registrar of any security held hereunder shall be required to inquire as to the propriety, validity or legality of any transfer made by the Trustee or such nominee.

F. 1. In the event that said _____ shall be unwilling or unable to continue to serve as Trustee hereunder, then, my _____, _____, of _____, _____, shall serve as successor Trustee hereunder. In the event that both said _____ and said _____ shall be unwilling or unable to serve or continue to serve as Trustee hereunder, then _____, of _____, _____, shall serve as successor Trustee hereunder. Any Trustee shall be entitled to resign as Trustee for any reason whatsoever by giving written notice to the Trustee designated to succeed it; provided that the Trustee designated to succeed it shall first execute a formal written acceptance of the duties and obligations of the Trustee hereunder and file an executed copy of such acceptance with the preceding Trustee. After this is done, and when all sums then due from the trust estate to such predecessor Trustee have been paid, such predecessor Trustee shall transfer the Trust property then in its hands to such successor Trustee and such predecessor Trustee shall thereupon and thereby be discharged of all subsequent duties and obligations under or arising out of its trusteeship.

2. Any successor Trustee shall have and enjoy all the powers, authorities, duties and immunities hereby vested in and imposed upon the original Trustee and no successor Trustee shall be obliged to inquire into or be in any way accountable for the previous administration of the trust property.

G. My Trustee is authorized, in its discretion, to sell to, purchase from, borrow funds from, lend funds to, or otherwise deal with, upon such terms and conditions as my Trustee shall deem just and equitable and for full and adequate consideration, the Executor of the Last Will and Testament of myself or my said **[wife/husband]** or the Trustee of any Trust established by me or my said **[wife/husband]** (whether such Trust is a testamentary or inter vivos trust), even though my Trustee may also be serving as Executor under my Will or my said **[wife/husband]**'s Will or as Trustee under any such Trust established by me or by my said **[wife/husband]**.

H. In determining the amount of any discretionary distributions of income or principal to a beneficiary of a trust created hereunder, the Trustee shall be required to take into account all other means and resources known to or reasonably ascertainable by the Trustee, including Medicaid or any other form of government assistance, which are available to such beneficiary for the purposes for which the Trustee is authorized to make said distributions.

I. _____, as Trustee, shall serve without compensation. Any other Trustee shall be entitled to receive reasonable compensation. Any Trustee shall be entitled to be reimbursed for reasonable expenses it incurs which are necessary to carry out its duties as Trustee hereunder.

J. No bond shall be required of the Trustee hereunder or any successor Trustee.

K. The Trustee and any successor Trustee are specifically instructed by the Settlor to maintain the privacy and confidentiality of this instrument and the trust created hereunder, and are in no circumstances to divulge its terms to any probate or other court or other public agency with the exception of a tax authority.

L. The Trustee and any successor Trustee shall have the authority to merge any trust held hereunder with any other trust, however created, which has similar provisions, the same beneficiaries and the same Trustee.

M. Notwithstanding any other provision contained herein, an individual Trustee (a) shall have no incident of ownership or power with respect to any policy of insurance upon such Trustee's life, and (b) shall have no power of discretion with respect to the allocation or distribution of assets to the extent that such would discharge such Trustee's legal obligation to support any beneficiary, or directly or indirectly benefit such Trustee unless necessary to provide for such Trustee's support in reasonable comfort, health care or education at any level, considering such Trustee's other financial resources.

ARTICLE VII
GOVERNING LAW

This Trust Agreement shall be construed under and in accordance with the laws of the State of _____.

IN WITNESS WHEREOF, I have hereunto set my hand, and the Trustee, to evidence its acceptance of the Trust herein expressed, has hereunto set its hand, in duplicate, at _____ _____, _____, on the day and year first above written.

Signed in the presence of:

_____   _____

_____   "Settlor"

_____   _____

_____   "Trustee"

I, the undersigned legal spouse of the Settlor, hereby waive all community property, dower or courtesy rights which I may have in the hereinabove-described property and give my assent to the provisions of the trust and to the inclusion in it of the said property.

_____

_____

Witness: _____   Witness: _____

STATE OF _____ City
or
COUNTY OF _____ Town _____

On the _____ day of _____, 19___, personally appeared
_____ known to me to be the individual(s) who executed the foregoing instrument, and acknowledged the same to be **[his/her]** free act and deed, before me.

_____
Notary Public

My commission expires:
_____

SCHEDULE A

The following is a true and correct Schedule A of the property assigned, delivered and conveyed to _____, Trustee, to be held, treated and disposed of in accordance with the terms of a certain Irrevocable Trust Agreement between _____, the Settlor, and _____, the Trustee, dated _____ ____, 19___, to which Agreement this Schedule A is attached and made a part thereof.

_____

_____

_____

_____

_____

_____

_____

_____

_____

_____

_____

_____

Signed in the presence of:

_____   _____

_____   _____
                                                                "Settlor"

_____   _____

_____   _____
                                                                "Trustee"

    I, the undersigned legal spouse of the Settlor, hereby waive all community property, dower or courtesy rights which I may have in the hereinabove-described property and give my assent to the provisions of the trust and to the inclusion in it of the said property.

                                         _____

                                         _____

Witness: _____   Witness: _____

_____   _____

9

ADDITION OF PROPERTY TO IRREVOCABLE TRUST AGREEMENT
BY _____
DATED _____ ___, 19___
WITH _____, TRUSTEE

_____ (the "Assignor"), pursuant to the terms of the above-described Irrevocable Trust Agreement, does hereby assign, transfer and convey to _____, Trustee, and _____ _____, Trustee, does hereby acknowledge receipt of, the following assets from the Assignor:

_____

_____

_____

_____

_____

_____

_____

_____

_____

_____

_____

_____

The Trustee agrees to hold, manage and administer the above assets as a part of the trust estate created under such Irrevocable Trust Agreement.

At the request of the Trustee, the Assignor shall fully cooperate and execute any and all documents deemed necessary or desirable by it in order to cause the assignment made hereby to be properly recorded.

IN WITNESS WHEREOF, the Assignor and the Trustee have signed their names at _____, _____, on this _____ day of _____, 19___.

Signed in the presence of:

_____   _____

_____   _____, Assignor

_____   _____

_____   _____, Trustee

10

I, the undersigned legal spouse of the Assignor, hereby waive all community property, dower or courtesy rights which I may have in the hereinabove-described property and give my assent to the inclusion in the trust of the said property.

_____

_____

Witness: _____   Witness: _____

STATE OF _____   City
                                     or
COUNTY OF _____   Town _____

On the _____ day of _____, 19___, personally appeared _____ known to me to be the individual(s) who executed the foregoing instrument, and acknowledged the same to be **[his/her]** free act and deed, before me.

_____
Notary Public

My commission expires:
_____

Medicaid Trust No. 2
For Individual Who Is Married, Keeping Assets in Trust for Children

Instructions/Explanation

As you can readily see, the trust agreement is filled with legalese. Don't be scared off by this confusing language. The explanations that follow should provide you with a clear understanding of the terms used.

Introduction: In the first blanks, fill in the city and state where you reside and the day, month, and year in which you are executing the Agreement.

Next, put in your name and residence (city and state)—the "Settlor" is your title when you make a trust. Then fill in the name, city, and state of the person or institution whom you are naming as trustee.

Remember, neither you nor your spouse should be the trustee. A child or other close relative will probably be your first choice (keeping in mind possible tax consequences where annual distributions of over $10,000 will be made). If no one fits that description, you may have to name an institutional trustee, such as a bank.

Article I(A): This is the section making your trust irrevocable. Once you sign the Agreement, you will never be able to change, amend, or revoke it.

Article I(B): This paragraph transfers into the Trust all the items listed on Schedule A at the end of the Agreement. You can include on Schedule A just about any item imaginable, including real estate, personal property, savings and checking accounts, boats, cars, even clothing.

If the property you put into the trust increases in value, the increased value is part of the trust. And if an asset changes form, the new asset still remains in the trust. For example, if the trustee takes $5,000 from a bank account and buys $5,000 worth of stock, the stock remains in the trust.

While you can never remove assets once they are placed into the trust, you can always add to the trust by using the Addition to Trust form following Schedule A.

A testamentary gift, referred to in this paragraph, is a gift given at the time of someone's death, normally contained in a will. For example, you may

not put your car into trust immediately, but you may add to your trust under your will when you die.

IMPORTANT NOTE: In Paragraph I(B) and throughout this Trust Agreement, you will see references to [wife/husband]. If your spouse is a female, strike out husband; if a male, strike out wife. On the line following [wife/husband], fill in the name.

Article II: This section gives you and your spouse the income from the trust during your lives, but specifically provides that you cannot get at the principal. This is *absolutely crucial* to saving your estate from the grasp of a nursing home if either you or your spouse enters one. With this language, Medicaid cannot require you to spend the principal on the nursing home *because you don't control or even have access to the principal.*

Why does the Trust Agreement give discretion to the Trustee to pay you and/or your spouse income rather than requiring the Trustee to pay all the income? Because with this provision, you *may* be able to protect your income from the nursing home.

Let's say the Trust Agreement just said that all the income was automatically yours. If you entered a nursing home, Medicaid would force you to pay all the income to the nursing home and would only cover any deficiency on the bill. But if the Trustee has discretion to pay all the income to you or your spouse, after you go into a nursing home the Trustee might decide to pay all the income to your spouse and none to you. In that situation, Medicaid might pay the entire nursing-home tab, because you don't have any income. (I say might because the law and its application to situations like this are not yet clear. It is possible that Medicaid might say that, even if you're not actually receiving any income, you *could* receive some or all of the income and so it won't pay the full nursing-home bill.)

Article III: This section describes how your trust principal, less any of your estate taxes, estate administration costs, or funeral expenses as provided in

Article VI(C) will be distributed after you and/or your spouse die.

Paragraph III(A)(1) provides that, if you die before your spouse, your spouse gets the income from the trust during his or her lifetime. Your spouse can't get at the principal during his or her life, so that if he or she goes into a nursing home, the principal will remain protected for your heirs.

Then when your spouse dies, Paragraph III(A)(2) says that the balance of your trust principal will be held, administered, and distributed pursuant to Paragraph III(B).

Paragraph III(B) says that, after you die, the balance of your trust principal will be split into equal shares for each of your children. If you have three children, all of whom are living at the time of your death, there will be three shares; if you had three children, one of whom has died, there will still be three shares, with the third share for your deceased child's children. Each share will continue to be held in trust until the death of each child, at which time the child's share will be disbursed to his or her children (your grandchildren). During the lifetime of each of your children, the income and principal from the child's share may be used for your child's benefit.

Why do this? There are two primary reasons you might want a trust like this. First, you may be able to save your children estate taxes. By leaving the principal in trust for your children, the principal is not in their estate when they die. Assuming your assets in the trust are under one million dollars, there is no generation-skipping tax. This may be primarily appealing if your children have or are likely to have large estates when they die.

The second reason for this provision is to keep principal from a child or children who may not be capable of adequately handling the funds.

Paragraph III(C) provides for the distribution of the trust if there's no one to receive the principal from your trust under Paragraphs III(A) or (B). If you and your spouse die leaving no living children or grandchildren, Paragraph III(C) takes over.

Under III(C), the remaining principal of the trust will be divided into two parts. One part will go to those persons who would inherit from you under the laws of your state as if you had died without a will or a trust. Every state has a law that dictates to whom an estate of someone who dies without a will will be distributed—usually to the closest living relative(s) of the deceased. For example, if you die

without children or grandchildren, Paragraph III(C) may mean that your parent or brother collects part of the trust estate.

The other half of the trust estate will be distributed to those persons who would inherit from your deceased spouse under the laws of your state as if he or she had died without a will.

The estate is split into two parts so that relatives on both sides of your family are treated equally. For example, rather than having everything go to your cousin, half may go to your cousin and half to your deceased spouse's sister.

Fill in the blanks in Paragraph III(C) with the name of your state.

Part III(D) discusses distributions, after you and your spouse die, to beneficiaries named in your trust who are under some legal disability or are unable to administer their distributions. For example, if your spouse is senile or suffering from Alzheimer's disease, he or she may be under a legal disability or unable to manage his or her money. Or if a distribution under your trust is to go to a young child (perhaps the children of a deceased child of yours), Part III(D) may come into play.

If a distribution from your trust is to go to someone who is under a legal disability or unable to manage their money, the Trustee has four options:

1. Pay the money to the beneficiary.
2. Make the distribution to a legal guardian of the beneficiary.
3. Distribute the beneficiary's portion to a custodian for the beneficiary.
4. Spend the money himself or herself for the benefit of the beneficiary.

If, when you make up your trust, you could predict the ages and physical and mental conditions of all your beneficiaries at the time of your death, you could spell out which of these four options you would want the Trustee to pursue. But since you can't, this Trust allows the Trustee to choose which option he or she believes is best.

The last sentence of Part III(D) says that, once the Trustee has made his or her choice and distributed a beneficiary's portion to the beneficiary or to the beneficiary's guardian or custodian, the Trustee is off the hook; he or she doesn't have to monitor the use of the distribution after that.

Part III(E), often called a spendthrift clause, provides that nobody but your intended beneficiary can obtain an interest in a distribution under your

Trust. For example, your child, who will receive a portion of your Trust after you're gone, can't sell his or her expected distribution in the future to someone for cash now. And a beneficiary can't put up his or her interest in a distribution as collateral for a loan. After all, you want the person you name in the Trust to receive a distribution, not some stranger.

Spendthrift clauses like this are enforced in most, but not all, states. If you have a serious concern that a beneficiary has or may have creditor problems, consult with a local attorney to determine whether this clause will be effective in your state.

Trusts cannot legally tie up assets forever, so Part III(F) is designed to avoid potential problems by limiting the life of the Trust.

Article IV: Let's say you and your spouse are killed in an accident together. One of you must have died minutes before the other. Rather than leave open the possibility of confusion over who died first, this paragraph says that your spouse will be considered to have died first.

Article V: This is the definition section. The only important point here is to recognize that a legally adopted child will be considered a child for purposes of the Trust Agreement. So by leaving everything to your children equally after you and your spouse die, any adopted child would be treated the same as a natural child.

Article VI: This section deals with the powers and duties you are giving to the Trustee.

Part VI(A) says that, after your death, the Trustee must collect the money due under any insurance policy on your life. The Trustee does not have a duty to pay your life insurance premiums during your lifetime, until and unless the Trustee takes title to any insurance policy.

Part VI(B) is very important, setting forth the powers of the Trustee. As you can see, this Trust Agreement gives the Trustee very broad powers to administer the funds and property in the estate, including the power to:

1. Buy real estate or personal property from your or your spouse's estate. Without this power, purchases by your Trustee from your estate at death might not be allowed.
2. Keep in the Trust anything received from you, your spouse, or your and your spouse's estates.
3. Sell, exchange, mortgage, and do just about anything else with property in the Trust.
4. Invest the assets in the Trust in just about anything.
5. Borrow money for the Trust.
6. Manage stock and other securities.
7. Collect money for the Trust.
8. Handle claims and lawsuits for or against the Trust.
9. Hire and pay counselors and assistants, like lawyers and accountants, for the Trust.
10. Hold property in his or her own name, in the name of a nominee, or in bearer form.
11. Manage real estate in the Trust, including repairing, improving, or converting property.
12. Handle life insurance policies in the Trust, including paying premiums, canceling or selling policies, cashing in policies, or borrowing against them.
13. Make distributions under the Trust in cash or in property.
14. Receive additional property for the Trust.
15. Do anything else reasonably required to manage, protect, or preserve the Trust assets.

Why put in many specific powers, instead of just having item 15, which generally allows the Trustee to do anything reasonably necessary? Because with only a general statement, someone with whom the Trustee must deal may question his or her power and may refuse to do business with him or her. For example, without specifically giving the Trustee the power to sell real estate, buyers, lenders, and escrow agents may be hesitant to deal with him or her, even if your trust agreement generally gives him or her broad powers. By listing specific powers, you can ensure the Trustee's ability properly to manage the Trust.

Why give the Trustee such broad powers anyway? Why not just specify a few actions he or she may take? The reason is simple: you can't predict what the Trustee may need to do to manage your estate properly, and if you don't give him or her broad powers, you may hamper him or her and damage your Trust estate. For example, if you don't own any stocks, why give the Trustee power to manage them? Because at some point it might be in your best interest for your Trustee to purchase securities and your Trust Agreement could unnecessarily prevent him or her from doing so.

Part VI(C) provides for certain payments from

your Trust upon your death. If the representative of your estate (such as the executor or administrator) decides that the funds left in your estate (not in your Trust) are insufficient to pay your estate taxes, expenses of administration, or funeral expenses, he or she can require the Trustee to cover those costs. The Trustee does not have to get anything in return, and your estate representative does not have to repay the money. Once the Trustee has paid the representative of your estate, the Trustee has no further obligation to monitor the use of these funds.

Part VI(D) requires the Trustee to keep accurate records showing all transactions in the Trust. Every year, the Trustee must give to certain beneficiaries a statement listing the Trust transactions for the year and a current inventory of assets in the Trust. Not every possible future beneficiary of the Trust gets this report. For example, if the Trust Agreement provides income to you for your lifetime, then on your death the assets will be distributed to your children or their children, only you are entitled to the Trustee's report.

Part VI(E) is designed to encourage people to deal with the Trustee by relieving them of liability in case the Trustee takes some action beyond his power. For example, if the Trustee attempts to sell a house, the buyer can go ahead with the transaction and pay the Trustee without worrying about whether the Trust really allows the Trustee to make that deal.

Part VI(F)(1) allows you to name alternative Trustees in case your first and/or second choice can't or won't serve when the time comes. In the first blank, put the name of your first choice for Trustee. In the next three blanks, fill in the relationship to you, the name and residence of your second choice. In the next two blanks, fill in the names of your first and second choices for Trustee. In the last three blanks, include the name, city, and state of a third choice for Trustee.

Part VI(F)(2) gives any successor Trustee all the same powers and duties as the original Trustee. It also encourages your chosen successor Trustee to accept the job by providing that he has no responsibility for anything done by the earlier Trustee.

Part VI(G) authorizes the Trustee to engage in transactions with the Executor of your or your spouse's estate or any trustee of any other trust established by you or your spouse. Without this language, a conflict-of-interest issue could arise over these types of dealings.

Part VI(H) concerns discretionary distributions by the Trustee. Under Article II, the Trustee is given discretion to distribute to you and your spouse all the net income of the trust. Let's say one of you enters a nursing home—will some or all of the income from the trust have to be paid to the nursing home? Under the law as it stands now, the answer is not totally clear. Medicaid may take the position that at least half and maybe *all* of the income must be paid to the nursing-home spouse (and so to the nursing home). But with Part VI(H), there is a chance you can save part or all of the income.

Under Part VI(H), the Trustee could decide to pay all the income to the spouse-at-home. In fact, by requiring the Trustee to consider other resources available, including Medicaid, you are tilting the Trustee's decision in the direction of your spouse. If the Trustee makes that decision, Medicaid might allow the outside spouse to retain the income while it pays the institutional spouse's costs.

In Part VI(I), you are providing that the Trustee (whose name must be filled in the blank) will serve without compensation. Since the Trustee will probably be your child or someone else close to you, that should be agreeable. Other possible trustees, such as a bank, will want to be paid, and Part VI(I) allows that as well.

Part VI(J) states that the Trustee does not have to post a bond. A bond is like an insurance policy, designed to protect your Trust in case the Trustee does something wrong, such as steals assets. Depending on the amount in the Trust, the bond could easily cost your Trust several hundred dollars. If you've followed the tips in this book and selected the right Trustee, you shouldn't need a bond.

Part VI(K) instructs the Trustee to keep the terms of your Trust private to the maximum extent possible. A trust has a great advantage over a will when it comes to passing your assets along after your death. Your estate becomes an open book when it goes through probate; when it passes under a trust, it can be kept from the eyes of nosy neighbors.

Part VI(L) allows the Trustee to merge trusts that are very similar to avoid duplication of effort and costs.

Part VI(M) is a protection for the Trustee to avoid the remote possibility of having the trust property included in the Trustee's estate, causing adverse tax consequences.

Article VII: Article VII states that any questions about the Trust will be answered by the laws of the state of your primary residence. In the blank space, fill in the name of your state.

Conclusion: In the blanks in the final paragraph, fill in your city and state. Then sign where it says Settlor (that's you) and have the Trustee sign below that. You and the Trustee should each print your names below the signature lines. To the left of your and the Trustee's signatures, two witnesses to each signature must sign. The witnesses can be the same, but they don't have to be; if they are the same, they must sign twice (once for the Settlor and once for the Trustee). The witnesses cannot be members of your family.

Then your spouse should also sign, and two witnesses must sign below. In many states, your spouse has a legal interest in your property and must waive his or her rights in writing to the property covered by the trust.

The final section is for a notary public.

Schedule A: Following the end of the Trust is Schedule A, on which you should list any items (i.e., cash accounts, real estate, personal property, etc.) to be placed under the control of the Trustee. Identify each item as best you can, using addresses, registration numbers, account numbers, etc., wherever possible, to avoid confusion.

On Schedule A, fill in: the name of the Trustee in the first blank, your name (the "Settlor") in the second blank, and the name of the Trustee again in the third blank. Then date the Schedule.

At the bottom, you, the Trustee, and your spouse should sign before two independent witnesses.

Addition of Property Form: Finally included is a form that you can use to add property to the Trust later. At the top, fill in your name, the date that the Trust was originally made, and the name of the Trustee. In the first full paragraph, fill in your name as the Assignor, assigning property to the Trustee. Then on the lines that follow, list any items to be added to the Trust. Again, identify each item as best you can. At the end, you, the Trustee, and your spouse should sign before two independent witnesses and a notary.

IRREVOCABLE TRUST AGREEMENT

THIS IRREVOCABLE TRUST AGREEMENT is entered into at _____
_____, _____, this _____ day of _____, 19__, by and
between _____ of _____,
_____, the Settlor, hereinafter referred to in the first person,
and _____, of _____,
_____, the Trustee, hereinafter referred to as the "Trustee" and
sometimes in the third person impersonal.

ARTICLE I

CREATION OF TRUST

A. Except as provided in Paragraph B of this Article I, this Trust Agreement shall be
irrevocable, and I hereby expressly acknowledge that I shall have no right or power, either alone or
in conjunction with others, and in any capacity whatsoever, to alter, amend, modify, revoke or terminate
this Trust or any of the terms of this Trust Agreement in whole or in part, or otherwise to cause any
of the assets of the Trust to revert to me or to my estate.

B. I hereby transfer the property listed in Schedule A of this Trust Agreement to the
Trustee. That property and all proceeds, investments and reinvestments thereof and any property
hereinafter received by the Trustee from me, my **[wife/husband]**, _____,
or from any other person (such property being hereinafter referred to as the "trust estate") shall be
held, administered and distributed in accordance with the terms of the trust herein expressed. I reserve
to myself and to others the right to add property to the trust estate by lifetime or testamentary gifts,
all of which added property shall be governed by the terms hereof.

ARTICLE II

DISTRIBUTIONS DURING LIFETIME OF SETTLOR

During my lifetime, the Trustee may distribute to or for the benefit of me or my
[wife/husband], _____, out of the net income of the trust estate, such amount or amounts
as the Trustee deems necessary to provide for my and/or my said **[wife's/husband's]** maintenance
and support. At the end of each taxable year the Trustee shall add any undistributed income to the
principal of the trust estate being held hereunder.

ARTICLE III

DIVISION OF TRUST ESTATE UPON SETTLOR'S DEATH

Upon my death, the Trustee shall hold, administer and distribute the property held
hereunder, as the same shall be constituted after being (a) augmented by property received or to be
received by the Trustee as a consequence of my death, including, without limitation, any property
received or to be received under the terms of my Last Will and Testament or any Codicil thereto and
(b) depleted by any money disbursed by the Trustee pursuant to the provisions of Paragraph C of
Article VI hereof (said property as so constituted being hereinafter referred to as "The Family Trust")
in accordance with the following provisions of this Trust Agreement.

1

A. Upon my death, if my **[wife/husband]**, _____, survives me:

1. During my said **[wife's/husband's]** lifetime, the Trustee may distribute to or for the benefit of my said **[wife/husband]** such amount or amounts of the net income of The Family Trust as the Trustee deems necessary to provide for my said **[wife's/husband's]** maintenance and support. At the end of each taxable year, the Trustee shall add any undistributed income to the principal of the trust estate being held hereunder.

2. Upon the death of my said **[wife/husband]**, the Trustee may pay to my said **[wife's/husband's]** estate cash and/or properties aggregating in value an amount or amounts requested in writing by the representative thereof, to pay and/or assist in satisfying my said **[wife's/husband's]** funeral expenses or the expenses of administration of **[her/his]** estate. The Trustee shall have no duty to ascertain or examine into the correctness of any amounts so requested, nor to see to the application of any funds paid over to **[her/his]** estate, the receipt of the representative thereof to be a complete acquittance to the Trustee hereunder with respect thereto. The balance of The Family Trust being held hereunder shall be distributed, subject to the provisions of Paragraph C of this Article III, to the following persons who survive me in the proportions shown, treating as a surviving person the then living collective issue of any such person who shall then be deceased, the distribution to such issue to be *per stirpes,* the root of the *per stirpes* distribution to be such predeceased person.

Name   *Proportion To Be Paid*

_____   _____%

_____   _____%

_____   _____%

_____   _____%

_____   _____%

_____   _____%

B. Upon my death if my said **[wife/husband]** does not survive me, the Trustee, subject to the provisions of Paragraph C of this Article III, shall distribute the balance of The Family Trust being held hereunder to the following persons who survive me in the proportions shown, treating as a surviving person the then living collective issue of any such person who shall then be deceased, the distribution to such issue to be *per stirpes,* the root of the *per stirpes* distribution to be such predeceased person.

Name   *Proportion To Be Paid*

_____   _____%

_____   _____%

_____   _____%

_____   _____%

_____   _____%

_____   _____%

C. If, under the provisions of Paragraphs A or B of this Article III, any portion of The Family Trust shall become distributable to any person who is then under the age of twenty-one (21) years, then such portion shall be retained by the Trustee in trust for the benefit of such person. The Trustee shall distribute to or for the benefit of such person out of the net income or principal or both of such portion held for such person, such amount or amounts (whether the whole or a lesser amount) as the Trustee, in its sole discretion, deems necessary or proper suitably to provide for the maintenance, support, health, and education of such person, and shall from time to time add to the principal of such portion the remaining undistributed income, if any, until such person shall attain the age of twenty-one (21) years, whereupon the Trustee shall distribute all of such portion to such person. If such person shall die prior to receiving the complete distribution of the portion held for such person's benefit, such portion shall be distributed free of the trust to such person's estate.

D. If at the time for distribution of The Family Trust or any share or portion of the trust estate being held pursuant to this Article III, there is no person or person's estate entitled under the provisions of this Article III other than this Paragraph D to take such distribution, the Trustee shall divide the trust estate into two (2) equal shares. One such share shall be distributed free of the trust to such person or persons as would be entitled to inherit from me and in the proportions they would so inherit under the laws of the State of _____ as though I had died intestate and domiciled in the State of _____ at the time distribution is so to be made. The other such share shall be distributed free of the trust to such person or persons as would be entitled to inherit from my said **[wife/husband]** and in the proportions they would so inherit under the laws of the State of _____ as though **[she/he]** had died intestate and domiciled in the State of _____ at the time distribution is so to be made.

E. If the Trustee is authorized pursuant to the provisions of this Article III to make distributions or payments to or for the benefit of any person (including distributions or payments directed or permitted to be made to a person who is under legal disability or, in the reasonable opinion of the Trustee, is unable properly to administer such distributions or payments), the Trustee may make such distributions or payments in any one or more of the following ways, as the Trustee may deem advisable: (1) directly to such beneficiary; (2) to the legal guardian of such beneficiary; (3) to any custodian then serving for such beneficiary, or to any person designated by the Trustee to serve as a custodian for such beneficiary (any such custodian may be the Trustee); or (4) by the Trustee itself expending such income or principal for the benefit of such beneficiary. The Trustee shall not be required to see to the application of any distribution or payment so made, but the receipt of any of the persons mentioned in Clause (1), (2) or (3) in the immediately preceding sentence shall be a full discharge for the Trustee.

F. All interests of a beneficiary hereunder shall be inalienable and free from anticipation, assignment, attachment, pledge or control by creditors or a present or former spouse of such beneficiary in any proceedings at law or in equity.

G. Any provisions of this Article III to the contrary notwithstanding, if not already distributed, all accrued and undistributed income and the entire principal of every trust estate then held hereunder shall be paid over and distributed outright and free of the trust not later than the end of the day immediately preceding the expiration of twenty-one (21) years from and after the death of the last survivor of myself, my said **[wife/husband]**, my children and my children's issue living at the time of the death of the first to die of my said **[wife/husband]** and me. Such payment and distribution shall be made to the person or persons for whose benefit the trust estate or estates respectively shall then be held hereunder.

ARTICLE IV

DETERMINATION OF SURVIVOR

If my **[wife/husband]**, _____, and I shall die under such circumstances that there is not sufficient evidence to determine the order of our deaths, or if **[she/he]** shall die within a period of thirty (30) days after the date of my death, then, for the purposes of this Trust Agreement, my said **[wife/husband]** shall be deemed not to have survived me.

ARTICLE V
DEFINITIONS

A. The words "issue," "child" and "children," as used herein, shall be deemed to include any legally adopted person as if he or she were the natural child of the adopting parent.

B. Whenever the context so requires, the use of words herein in the singular shall be construed to include the plural, and words in the plural, the singular, and words whether in the masculine, feminine or neuter gender shall be construed to include all of said genders.

ARTICLE VI
POWERS AND DUTIES OF THE TRUSTEE

A. There shall be no duty on the Trustee to pay or see to the payment of any premiums on any policies of life insurance or to take any steps to keep them in force, until such time as the Trustee holds title to any insurance policies hereunder as a part of the corpus of any trust estate. The Trustee furthermore assumes no responsibility with respect to the validity or enforceability of said policies. However, as soon as practicable after receiving notice of the death of the insured under any of such policies, the Trustee shall proceed to collect all amounts payable thereunder. The Trustee shall have full and complete authority to collect and receive any and all such amounts and its receipt therefor shall be a full and complete acquittance to any insurer or payor, who shall be under no obligation to see to the proper application thereof by the Trustee.

B. In the administration of the trusts created hereunder and in addition to the powers exercised by trustees generally, the Trustee shall have the following powers and authorities without any court order or proceeding, exercisable in the discretion of the Trustee:

1. To purchase as an investment for the trust estate or estates any property, real or personal, belonging to my estate and/or the estate of my **[wife/husband]**, _____;

2. To retain as suitable investments for the trust estate or estates any properties (including, without limitation, securities issued by any corporate Trustee or the holding company of which it is an affiliate) received by it from me, my said **[wife/husband]**, my estate and/or the estate of my said **[wife/husband]**, and whether received by purchase or in any other manner, without regard to any law, statutory or judicial, or any rule or practice of court now or hereafter in force specifying or limiting the permissible investments of trustees, trust companies or fiduciaries generally or requiring the diversification of investments, and without liability to any person whomsoever for loss or depreciation in value thereof;

3. To sell, exchange, convey, mortgage, pledge, lease, control, and manage, and to make contracts concerning, any of the properties, real or personal, comprised in the trust estate or estates, all either publicly or privately and for such considerations and upon such terms as to credit or otherwise as may be reasonable under the circumstances, which leases and contracts may extend beyond the duration of any of the trusts created hereunder; to give options therefor; and to execute deeds, transfers, mortgages, leases and other instruments of any kind;

4. To invest and reinvest the properties from time to time comprised in the trust estate or estates in stocks, common and/or preferred, bonds, notes, debentures, loans, mortgages, common trust funds, or other securities or property, real or personal, all limitations now or hereafter imposed by law, statutory or judicial, or by any rule or practice of court now or hereafter in force specifying or limiting the permissible investments of trustees, trust companies or fiduciaries generally or

requiring the diversification of investments, being hereby expressly waived, it being the intent hereof that the Trustee shall have full power and authority to deal with the trust estate or estates in all respects as though it was the sole owner thereof, without order of court or other authority;

5. To borrow money, from itself or otherwise, with or without security, whenever it deems such action advisable;

6. To exercise voting rights, execute and deliver powers of attorney and proxies and similarly act with reference to shares of stock and other securities comprised in the trust estate or estates in such manner as it deems proper, including, without limitation, the power to participate in or oppose reorganizations, recapitalizations, mergers, consolidations, exchanges, liquidations, arrangements and other corporate actions;

7. To collect all money; in accordance with generally accepted trust accounting principles, to determine whether money or other property coming into its possession shall be treated as principal or income and to charge or apportion expenses, taxes, gains and losses to principal or income;

8. To compromise, adjust and settle claims in favor of or against the trust estate or estates upon such terms and conditions as it may deem best; in the case of any litigation in connection with any part of such trust estate or estates, it may, under advice of its counsel, arbitrate, settle, or adjust any such matter in dispute upon such terms as it may consider just and equitable, and its decision shall be binding upon the beneficiaries;

9. To employ investment counsel, custodians of estate property, brokers, accountants, attorneys, clerical or bookkeeping assistants, and other suitable agents and to pay their reasonable compensation and expenses in addition to any compensation payable to the Trustee, and to execute and deliver powers of attorney; the Trustee shall not be liable for any neglect, omission or wrongdoing of such investment counsel, custodians, brokers, accountants, attorneys, assistants or agents, provided reasonable care shall have been exercised in their selection;

10. To hold title to stocks, bonds, or other securities or property, real or personal, in its own name or in the name of its nominee and without indication of any fiduciary capacity or to hold any such bonds or securities in bearer form; the Trustee shall assume full responsibility for the acts of any nominee selected by it;

11. To make all repairs, alterations or improvements of any real property which shall constitute a part of the trust estate or estates; adjust boundaries thereof, and to erect or demolish buildings thereon; and, with respect to such property, to convert for different use, grant easements for adequate consideration, partition, and insure for any or all risks;

12. To pay premiums on any policies of life insurance which may form a part of the trust estate or estates; to cancel, sell, assign, hypothecate, pledge or otherwise dispose of any of said policies; to exercise any right, election, option or privilege granted by any of said policies; to borrow any sums in accordance with the provisions of any of said policies, and to receive all payments, dividends, surrender values, additions, benefits or privileges of any kind which may accrue to any of said policies;

13. To make any allocation, division or distribution required or permitted hereunder in cash or in kind, in real or personal property, or an undivided interest therein, or partly in cash and partly in kind, and to do so without making pro rata allocations, divisions or distributions of specific assets, property allocated, divided or distributed in kind to be taken at its fair market value at the time of such allocation, division or distribution;

14. To receive, in accordance with the provisions of Article I hereof, additional property from me or any other person, the Trustee being authorized and empowered to merge and hold as one any duplicate trusts held for the same beneficiary;

15. To make such expenditures and do such other acts as are reasonably required to manage, improve, protect, preserve, invest or sell any of the trust estates or otherwise properly to administer this Trust.

C. If the representative of my estate, in such representative's sole discretion, shall determine that appropriate assets of my estate are not available in sufficient amount to pay (a) taxes levied against or with respect to my taxable estate by reason of my death, including interest and penalties thereon, if any, and (b) expenses of administration of my estate, the Trustee shall, upon the request of the representative of my estate, contribute from the principal of the trust estate the amount of such deficiency; and in connection with any such action the Trustee shall rely upon the written statement of the representative of my estate as to the validity and correctness of the amounts of any such taxes, expenses and bequests, and shall furnish funds to such representative so as to enable such representative to discharge the same, or to discharge any part or all thereof themselves by making payment directly to the governmental official or agency or to the person entitled or claiming to be entitled to receive payment thereof. No consideration need be required by the Trustee from the representative of my estate for any disbursement made by the Trustee pursuant hereto, nor shall there be any obligation upon such representative to repay to the Trustee any of the funds disbursed by it hereunder, and all amounts disbursed by the Trustee pursuant to the authority hereby conferred upon it shall be disbursed without any right in or duty upon the Trustee to seek or obtain contribution or reimbursement from any person or property on account of such payment. The Trustee shall not be responsible for the application of any funds delivered by it to the representative of my estate pursuant to the authority herein granted, nor shall the Trustee be subject to liability to any beneficiary hereunder on account of any payment made by it pursuant to the provisions hereof.

D. The Trustee shall keep accurate records showing all receipts and disbursements and other transactions involving the trust estate or estates and shall furnish annually to each beneficiary currently entitled to income, (1) a statement of the receipts and disbursements affecting such beneficiary's interest in the trust, and (2) a complete inventory of the trust estate then held for the benefit of such beneficiary.

E. No person, firm or corporation dealing with the Trustee or a nominee of the Trustee or performing any act pursuant to action taken or order given by the Trustee or such nominee shall be obliged to inquire as to the propriety, validity or legality thereof hereunder, nor shall any such person be liable for the application of any money or other consideration paid to the Trustee or such nominee, but, instead, may rely upon any action taken by the Trustee or such nominee pursuant to the powers and authorities conferred upon it under the provisions of this Article VI in all respects as if the same were completely unlimited. No transfer agent or registrar of any security held hereunder shall be required to inquire as to the propriety, validity or legality of any transfer made by the Trustee or such nominee.

F. 1. In the event that said _____ shall be unwilling or unable to continue to serve as Trustee hereunder, then, my _____, _____, of _____, _____, shall serve as successor Trustee hereunder. In the event that both said _____ and said _____ shall be unwilling or unable to serve or continue to serve as Trustee hereunder, then _____, of _____, _____, shall serve as successor Trustee hereunder. Any Trustee shall be entitled to resign as Trustee for any reason whatsoever by giving written notice to the Trustee designated to succeed it; provided that the Trustee designated to succeed it shall first execute a formal written acceptance of the duties and obligations of the Trustee hereunder and file an executed copy of such acceptance with the preceding Trustee. After this is done, and when all sums then due from the trust

6

estate to such predecessor Trustee have been paid, such predecessor Trustee shall transfer the Trust property then in its hands to such successor Trustee and such predecessor Trustee shall thereupon and thereby be discharged of all subsequent duties and obligations under or arising out of its trusteeship.

2. Any successor Trustee shall have and enjoy all the powers, authorities, duties and immunities hereby vested in and imposed upon the original Trustee and no successor Trustee shall be obliged to inquire into or be in any way accountable for the previous administration of the trust property.

G. My Trustee is authorized, in its discretion, to sell to, purchase from, borrow funds from, lend funds to, or otherwise deal with, upon such terms and conditions as my Trustee shall deem just and equitable and for full and adequate consideration, the Executor of the Last Will and Testament of myself or my said **[wife/husband]** or the Trustee of any Trust established by me or my said **[wife/husband]** (whether such Trust is a testamentary or inter vivos trust), even though my Trustee may also be serving as Executor under my Will or my said **[wife/husband]**'s Will or as Trustee under any such Trust established by me or by my said **[wife/husband]**.

H. In determining the amount of any discretionary distributions of income or principal to a beneficiary of a trust created hereunder, the Trustee shall be required to take into account all other means and resources known to or reasonably ascertainable by the Trustee, including Medicaid or any other form of government assistance, which are available to such beneficiary for the purposes for which the Trustee is authorized to make said distributions.

I. _____, as Trustee, shall serve without compensation. Any other Trustee shall be entitled to receive reasonable compensation. Any Trustee shall be entitled to be reimbursed for reasonable expenses it incurs which are necessary to carry out its duties as Trustee hereunder.

J. No bond shall be required of the Trustee hereunder or any successor Trustee.

K. The Trustee and any successor Trustee are specifically instructed by the Settlor to maintain the privacy and confidentiality of this instrument and the trust created hereunder, and are in no circumstances to divulge its terms to any probate or other court or other public agency with the exception of a tax authority.

L. The Trustee and any successor Trustee shall have the authority to merge any trust held hereunder with any other trust, however created, which has similar provisions, the same beneficiaries and the same Trustee.

M. Notwithstanding any other provision contained herein, an individual Trustee (a) shall have no incident of ownership or power with respect to any policy of insurance upon such Trustee's life, and (b) shall have no power of discretion with respect to the allocation or distribution of assets to the extent that such would discharge such Trustee's legal obligation to support any beneficiary, or directly or indirectly benefit such Trustee unless necessary to provide for such Trustee's support in reasonable comfort, health care or education at any level, considering such Trustee's other financial resources.

ARTICLE VII

GOVERNING LAW

This Trust Agreement shall be construed under and in accordance with the laws of the State of _____.

IN WITNESS WHEREOF, I have hereunto set my hand, and the Trustee, to evidence its acceptance of the Trust herein expressed, has hereunto set its hand, in duplicate, at _____ _____, _____, _____, on the day and year first above written.

Signed in the presence of:

_____

_____   _____

_____   _____

                                                                        "Settlor"

_____   _____

_____   _____

                                                                        "Trustee"

       I, the undersigned legal spouse of the Settlor, hereby waive all community property, dower or courtesy rights which I may have in the hereinabove-described property and give my assent to the provisions of the trust and to the inclusion in it of the said property.

                                                    _____

                                                    _____

Witness: _____   Witness: _____

STATE OF _____   City
                                                                          or
COUNTY OF _____   Town _____

       On the _____ day of _____, 19___, personally appeared _____ known to me to be the individual(s) who executed the foregoing instrument, and acknowledged the same to be **[his/her]** free act and deed, before me.

                                                    _____
                                                    Notary Public

My commission expires:

_____

SCHEDULE A

The following is a true and correct Schedule A of the property assigned, delivered and conveyed to _____, Trustee, to be held, treated and disposed of in accordance with the terms of a certain Irrevocable Trust Agreement between _____, the Settlor, and _____, the Trustee, dated _____ ____, 19___, to which Agreement this Schedule A is attached and made a part thereof.

_____

_____

_____

_____

_____

_____

_____

_____

_____

_____

_____

_____

_____

_____

_____

Signed in the presence of:

_____

_____   _____
                                                                    "Settlor"

_____

_____   _____
                                                                    "Trustee"

I, the undersigned legal spouse of the Settlor, hereby waive all community property, dower or courtesy rights which I may have in the hereinabove-described property and give my assent to the provisions of the trust and to the inclusion in it of the said property.

_____

_____

Witness: _____   Witness: _____

_____   _____

9

ADDITION OF PROPERTY TO IRREVOCABLE TRUST AGREEMENT

BY _____

DATED _____ ___, 19___

WITH _____, TRUSTEE

_____ (the "Assignor"), pursuant to the terms of the above-described Irrevocable Trust Agreement, does hereby assign, transfer and convey to ___, Trustee, and _____ _____, Trustee, does hereby acknowledge receipt of, the following assets from the Assignor:

_____

_____

_____

_____

_____

_____

_____

_____

_____

_____

_____

_____

_____

_____

_____

_____

_____

The Trustee agrees to hold, manage and administer the above assets as a part of the trust estate created under such Irrevocable Trust Agreement.

At the request of the Trustee, the Assignor shall fully cooperate and execute any and all documents deemed necessary or desirable by it in order to cause the assignment made hereby to be properly recorded.

IN WITNESS WHEREOF, the Assignor and the Trustee have signed their names at _____, _____, on this ___ day of _____, 19___.

Signed in the presence of:

_____   _____

_____   _____, Assignor

_____

_____   _____, Trustee

10

I, the undersigned legal spouse of the Assignor, hereby waive all community property, dower or courtesy rights which I may have in the hereinabove-described property and give my assent to the inclusion in the trust of the said property.

_____

_____

Witness: _____   Witness: _____

STATE OF _____   City
                                     or
COUNTY OF _____   Town _____

On the _____ day of _____, 19___, personally appeared
_____ known to me to be the individual(s) who executed the foregoing instrument, and acknowledged the same to be **[his/her]** free act and deed, before me.

_____
Notary Public

My commission expires:

_____

Medicaid Trust No. 3
for Individual Who Is Married, Distributing Assets After Death of Both Spouses to Children (Unequally) and/or to Others

Instructions/Explanation

As you can readily see, the trust agreement is filled with legalese. Don't be scared off by this confusing language. The explanations that follow should provide you with a clear understanding of the terms used.

Introduction: In the first blanks, fill in the city and state where you reside and the day, month, and year in which you are executing the Agreement.

Next, put in your name and residence (city and state)—the "Settlor" is your title when you make a trust. Then fill in the name, city, and state of the person or institution whom you are naming as trustee.

Remember, neither you nor your spouse should be the trustee. A child or other close relative will probably be your first choice (keeping in mind possible tax consequences where annual distributions of over $10,000 will be made). If no one fits that description, you may have to name an institutional trustee, such as a bank.

Article I(A): This is the section making your trust irrevocable. Once you sign the Agreement, you will never be able to change, amend, or revoke it.

Article I(B): This paragraph transfers into the Trust all the items listed on Schedule A at the end of the Agreement. You can include on Schedule A just about any item imaginable, including real estate, personal property, savings and checking accounts, boats, cars, even clothing.

If the property you put into the trust increases in value, the increased value is part of the trust. And if an asset changes form, the new asset still remains in the trust. For example, if the trustee takes $5,000 from a bank account and buys $5,000 worth of stock, the stock remains in the trust.

While you can never remove assets once they are placed into the trust, you can always add to the trust by using the Addition to Trust form following Schedule A.

A testamentary gift, referred to in this paragraph, is a gift given at the time of someone's death, normally contained in a will. For example, you may not put your car into trust immediately, but you may add to your trust under your will when you die.

IMPORTANT NOTE: In Paragraph I(B) and throughout this Trust Agreement, you will see references to [wife/husband]. If your spouse is a female, strike out husband; if a male, strike out wife. On the line following [wife/husband], fill in the name.

Article II: This section gives you and your spouse the income from the trust during your lives, but specifically provides that you cannot get at the principal. This is *absolutely crucial* to saving your estate from the grasp of a nursing home if either you or your spouse enters one. With this language, Medicaid cannot require you to spend the principal on the nursing home *because you don't control or even have access to the principal.*

Why does the Trust Agreement give discretion to the Trustee to pay you and/or your spouse income rather than requiring the Trustee to pay all the income? Because with this provision, you *may* be able to protect your income from the nursing home.

Let's say the Trust Agreement just said that all the income was automatically yours. If you entered a nursing home, Medicaid would force you to pay all the income to the nursing home and would only cover any deficiency on the bill. But if the Trustee has discretion to pay all the income to you or your spouse, after you go into a nursing home the Trustee might decide to pay all the income to your spouse and none to you. In that situation, Medicaid might pay the entire nursing-home tab, because you don't have any income. (I say might because the law and its application to situations like this are not yet clear. It is possible that Medicaid might say that, even if you're not actually receiving any income, you *could* receive some or all of the income and so it won't pay the full nursing-home bill.)

Article III: This section describes how your trust principal, less any of your estate taxes, estate administration costs, or funeral expenses as provided in Article VI(C), will be distributed after you and/or your spouse die.

Paragraph III(A)(1) provides that, if you die before your spouse, your spouse gets the income from the trust during his or her lifetime. Your spouse can't get at the principal during his or her life, so that if he or she goes into a nursing home, the principal will remain protected for your heirs.

When your spouse dies, Paragraph III(A)(2) says that the balance of your trust principal will be distributed to the persons you list in the Trust in the proportions you set. You can name anyone you choose: children, other family members, friends. You can also fix whatever percentages you wish; just make sure the percentages add up exactly to 100%. If any person named in the Trust has died before your spouse passed away, that person's portion goes to that person's children. A trust alternatively could provide that a deceased beneficiary's portion would be divided among the then-living named beneficiaries; if you'd prefer that arrangement, have your lawyer revise this section.

Paragraph III(B) provides for the distribution of the trust principal if you die after your spouse. The distribution should be the same as under III(A)(2), to the same persons and in the same proportions.

Paragraph III(C) provides that, if any person who is to receive a distribution is under age twenty-one, that person's distribution shall be kept in trust until that person reaches age twenty-one. This provision allows you to make sure that, if you have a young child or grandchild who is to receive a distribution from your trust, that child cannot have control of the funds until he or she is old enough (and, it is hoped, mature enough) to manage those funds. This trust provides for distribution of a child's portion upon reaching age twenty-one, although any age could be chosen and inserted into the trust.

Paragraph III(D) provides for the distribution of the trust if there's no one to receive the principal from your trust under Paragraphs III(A) or (B).

Under III(D), the remaining principal of the trust will be divided into two parts. One part will go to those persons who would inherit from you under the laws of your state as if you had died without a will or a trust. Every state has a law that dictates to whom an estate of someone who dies without a will will be distributed—usually to the closest living relative(s) of the deceased. For example, if you die without children or grandchildren, Paragraph III(D) may mean that your parent or brother collects part of the trust estate.

The other half of the trust estate will be distributed to those persons who would inherit from your deceased spouse under the laws of your state as if he or she had died without a will.

The estate is split into two parts so that relatives on both sides of your family are treated equally. For example, rather than having everything go to your cousin, half may go to your cousin and half to your deceased spouse's sister.

Fill in the blanks in Paragraph III(D) with the name of your state.

Part III(E) discusses distributions, after you die, to beneficiaries named in your trust who are under some legal disability or are unable to administer their distributions. For example, if your spouse is senile or suffering from Alzheimer's disease, he or she may be under a legal disability or unable to manage his or her money.

If a distribution from your trust is to go to someone who is under a legal disability or unable to manage their money, the Trustee has four options:

1. Pay the money to the beneficiary.
2. Make the distribution to a legal guardian of the beneficiary.
3. Distribute the beneficiary's portion to a custodian for the beneficiary.
4. Spend the money himself or herself for the benefit of the beneficiary.

If, when you make up your trust, you could predict the ages and physical and mental conditions of all your beneficiaries at the time of your death, you could spell out which of these four options you would want the Trustee to pursue. But since you can't, this Trust allows the Trustee to choose which option he or she believes is best.

The last sentence of Part III(E) says that, once the Trustee has made his or her choice and distributed a beneficiary's portion to the beneficiary or to the beneficiary's guardian or custodian, the Trustee is off the hook; he or she doesn't have to monitor the use of the distribution after that.

Part III(F), often called a spendthrift clause, provides that nobody but your intended beneficiary can obtain an interest in a distribution under your Trust. For example, your child, who may receive a portion of your Trust after you're gone, can't sell his or her expected distribution in the future to someone for cash now. And a beneficiary can't put up his or her interest in a distribution as collateral for a loan. After all, you want the person you name in the Trust to receive a distribution, not some stranger.

Spendthrift clauses like this are enforced in most, but not all, states. If you have a serious concern that a beneficiary has or may have creditor problems, consult with a local attorney to determine whether this clause will be effective in your state.

Trusts cannot legally tie up assets forever, so Part III(G) is designed to avoid potential problems by limiting the life of the Trust.

Article IV: Let's say you and your spouse are killed in an accident together. One of you must have died minutes before the other. Rather than leave open the possibility of confusion over who died first, this paragraph says that your spouse will be considered to have died first.

Article V: This is the definition section. The only important point here is to recognize that a legally adopted child will be considered a child for purposes of the Trust Agreement.

Article VI: This section deals with the powers and duties you are giving to the Trustee.

Part VI(A) says that, after your death, the Trustee must collect the money due under any insurance policy on your life. The Trustee does not have a duty to pay your life insurance premiums during your lifetime, until and unless the Trustee takes title to any insurance policy.

Part VI(B) is very important, setting forth the powers of the Trustee. As you can see, this Trust Agreement gives the Trustee very broad powers to administer the funds and property in the estate, including the power to:

1. Buy real estate or personal property from your or your spouse's estate. Without this power, purchases by your Trustee from your estate at death might not be allowed.
2. Keep in the Trust anything received from you, your spouse, or your and your spouse's estates.
3. Sell, exchange, mortgage, and do just about anything else with property in the Trust.
4. Invest the assets in the Trust in just about anything.
5. Borrow money for the Trust.
6. Manage stock and other securities.
7. Collect money for the Trust.
8. Handle claims and lawsuits for or against the Trust.
9. Hire and pay counselors and assistants, like lawyers and accountants, for the Trust.
10. Hold property in his or her own name, in the name of a nominee, or in bearer form.
11. Manage real estate in the Trust, including repairing, improving, or converting property.
12. Handle life insurance policies in the Trust, including paying premiums, cancelling or selling policies, cashing in policies, or borrowing against them.
13. Make distributions under the Trust in cash or in property.
14. Receive additional property for the Trust.
15. Do anything else reasonably required to manage, protect, or preserve the Trust assets.

Why put in many specific powers, instead of just having item 15, which generally allows the Trustee to do anything reasonably necessary? Because with only a general statement, someone with whom the Trustee must deal may question his or her power and may refuse to do business with him or her. For example, without specifically giving the Trustee the power to sell real estate, buyers, lenders, and escrow agents may be hesitant to deal with him or her, even if your trust agreement generally gives him or her broad powers. By listing specific powers, you can ensure the Trustee's ability properly to manage the Trust.

Why give the Trustee such broad powers anyway? Why not just specify a few actions he or she may take? The reason is simple: you can't predict what the Trustee may need to do to manage your estate properly, and if you don't give him or her broad powers, you may hamper him or her and damage your Trust estate. For example, if you don't own any stocks, why give the Trustee power to manage them? Because at some point it might be in your best interest for your Trustee to purchase securities, and your Trust Agreement could unnecessarily prevent him or her from doing so.

Part VI(C) provides for certain payments from your Trust upon your death. If the representative of your estate (such as the executor or administrator) decides that the funds left in your estate (not in your Trust) are insufficient to pay your estate taxes, expenses of administration, or funeral expenses, he or she can require the Trustee to cover those costs. The Trustee does not have to get anything in return, and your estate representative does not have to repay the money. Once the Trustee has paid the representative of your estate, the Trustee has no further obligation to monitor the use of these funds.

Part VI(D) requires the Trustee to keep accurate records showing all transactions in the Trust. Every year, the Trustee must give to certain beneficiaries a statement listing the Trust transactions for the year and a current inventory of assets in the Trust. Not every possible future beneficiary of the Trust gets this report. For example, if the Trust Agreement provides income to you for your lifetime, then on your death the assets will be distributed to your children or their children, only you are entitled to the Trustee's report.

Part VI(E) is designed to encourage people to deal with the Trustee by relieving them of liability in case the Trustee takes some action beyond his power. For example, if the Trustee attempts to sell a house, the buyer can go ahead with the transaction and pay the Trustee without worrying about whether the Trust really allows the Trustee to make that deal.

Part VI(F)(1) allows you to name alternative Trustees in case your first and/or second choice can't or won't serve when the time comes. In the first blank, put the name of your first choice for Trustee. In the next three blanks, fill in the relationship to you, the name and residence of your second choice. In the next two blanks, fill in the names of your first and second choices for Trustee. In the last three blanks, include the name, city, and state of a third choice for Trustee.

Part VI(F)(2) gives any successor Trustee all the same powers and duties as the original Trustee. It also encourages your chosen successor Trustee to accept the job by providing that he or she has no responsibility for anything done by the earlier Trustee.

Part VI(G) authorizes the Trustee to engage in transactions with the Executor of your or your spouse's estate or any trustee of any other trust established by you or your spouse. Without this language, a conflict-of-interest issue could arise over these types of dealings.

Part VI(H) concerns discretionary distributions by the Trustee. Under Article II, the Trustee is given discretion to distribute to you and your spouse all the net income of the trust. Let's say one of you enters a nursing home—will some or all of the income from the trust have to be paid to the nursing home? Under the law as it stands now, the answer is not totally clear. Medicaid may take the position that at least half and maybe *all* of the income must be paid to the nursing-home spouse (and so to the nursing home). But with Part VI(H), there is a chance you can save part or all of the income.

Under Part VI(H), the Trustee could decide to pay all the income to the spouse-at-home. In fact, by requiring the Trustee to consider other resources available, including Medicaid, you are tilting the Trustee's decision in the direction of your spouse. If the Trustee makes that decision, Medicaid might allow the outside spouse to retain the income while it pays the institutional spouse's costs.

In Part VI(I), you are providing that the Trustee (whose name must be filled in the blank) will serve without compensation. Since the Trustee will probably be your child or someone else close to you, that should be agreeable. Other possible trustees, such as a bank, will want to be paid, and Part VI(I) allows that as well.

Part VI(J) states that the Trustee does not have to post a bond. A bond is like an insurance policy, designed to protect your Trust in case the Trustee does something wrong, such as steals assets. Depending on the amount in the Trust, the bond could easily cost your Trust several hundred dollars. If you've followed the tips in this book and selected the right Trustee, you shouldn't need a bond.

Part VI(K) instructs the Trustee to keep the terms of your Trust private to the maximum extent possible. A trust has a great advantage over a will when it comes to passing your assets along after your death. Your estate becomes an open book when it goes through probate; when it passes under a trust, it can be kept from the eyes of nosy neighbors.

Part VI(L) allows the Trustee to merge trusts that are very similar to avoid duplication of effort and costs.

Part VI(M) is a protection for the Trustee to avoid the remote possibility of having the trust property included in the Trustee's estate, causing adverse tax consequences.

Article VII: Article VII states that any questions about the Trust will be answered by the laws of the state of your primary residence. In the blank space, fill in the name of your state.

Conclusion: In the blanks in the final paragraph, fill in your city and state. Then sign where it says Settlor (that's you) and have the Trustee sign below that. You and the Trustee should each print your names below the signature lines. To the left of your and the Trustee's signatures, two witnesses to each signature must sign. The witnesses can be the same, but they don't have to be; if they are the same, they must sign twice (once for the Settlor and once for the Trustee). The witnesses cannot be members of your family.

Then your spouse should also sign, and two witnesses must sign below. In many states, your spouse has a legal interest in your property and must waive his or her rights in writing to the property covered by the trust.

The final section is for a notary public.

Schedule A: Following the end of the Trust is Schedule A, on which you should list any items (i.e., cash accounts, real estate, personal property, etc.) to be placed under the control of the Trustee. Identify each item as best you can, using addresses, regis-

tration numbers, account numbers, etc., wherever possible, to avoid confusion.

On Schedule A, fill in: the name of the Trustee in the first blank, your name (the "Settlor") in the second blank, and the name of the Trustee again in the third blank. Then date the Schedule.

At the bottom, you, the Trustee, and your spouse should sign before two independent witnesses.

Addition of Property Form: Finally included is a form that you can use to add property to the Trust later. At the top, fill in your name, the date that the Trust was originally made, and the name of the Trustee. In the first full paragraph, fill in your name as the Assignor, assigning property to the Trustee. Then on the lines that follow, list any items to be added to the Trust. Again, identify each item as best you can. At the end, you, the Trustee, and your spouse should sign before two independent witnesses and a notary.

IRREVOCABLE TRUST AGREEMENT

THIS IRREVOCABLE TRUST AGREEMENT is entered into at _____
_____, _____, this _____ day of _____, 19__, by and
between _____, of _____,
_____, the Settlor, hereinafter referred to in the first person,
and _____, of _____,
_____, the Trustee, hereinafter referred to as the "Trustee" and
sometimes in the third person impersonal.

ARTICLE I

CREATION OF TRUST

A. Except as provided in Paragraph B of this Article I, this Trust Agreement shall be irrevocable, and I hereby expressly acknowledge that I shall have no right or power, either alone or in conjunction with others, and in any capacity whatsoever, to alter, amend, modify, revoke or terminate this Trust or any of the terms of this Trust Agreement in whole or in part, or otherwise to cause any of the assets of the Trust to revert to me or to my estate.

B. I hereby transfer the property listed in Schedule A of this Trust Agreement to the Trustee. That property and all proceeds, investments and reinvestments thereof and any property hereinafter received by the Trustee from me or from any other person (such property being herein-after referred to as the "trust estate") shall be held, administered and distributed in accordance with the terms of the trust herein expressed. I reserve to myself and to others the right to add property to the trust estate by lifetime or testamentary gifts, all of which added property shall be governed by the terms hereof.

ARTICLE II

DISTRIBUTIONS DURING LIFETIME OF SETTLOR

During my lifetime, the Trustee may distribute to or for the benefit of me, out of the net income of the trust estate, such amount or amounts as the Trustee deems necessary to provide for my maintenance and support. At the end of each taxable year the Trustee shall add any undistributed income to the principal of the trust estate being held hereunder.

ARTICLE III

DIVISION OF TRUST ESTATE UPON SETTLOR'S DEATH

Upon my death, the Trustee shall hold, administer and distribute the property held hereunder, as the same shall be constituted after being (a) augmented by property received or to be received by the Trustee as a consequence of my death, including, without limitation, any property received or to be received under the terms of my Last Will and Testament or any Codicil thereto and (b) depleted by any money disbursed by the Trustee pursuant to the provisions of Paragraph C of Article VI hereof (said property as so constituted being hereinafter referred to as "The Family Trust") in accordance with the following provisions of this Trust Agreement.

A. Upon my death, the Trustee shall distribute the balance of The Family Trust being held hereunder, in equal shares, to my children who survive me, treating as a surviving child of mine the then living collective issue of any child of mine who shall then be deceased, the distribution to such issue to be *per stirpes*, the root of the *per stirpes* distribution to be such predeceased child.

B. If at the time for distribution of The Family Trust or any share or portion of the trust estate being held pursuant to this Article III, there is no person or person's estate entitled under the provisions of this Article III other than this Paragraph B to take such distribution, the Trustee shall divide the trust estate into two (2) equal shares. One such share shall be distributed free of the trust to such person or persons as would be entitled to inherit from me and in the proportions they would so inherit under the laws of the State of _____ as though I had died intestate and domiciled in the State of _____ at the time distribution is so to be made. The other such share shall be distributed free of the trust to such person or persons as would be entitled to inherit from my deceased **[wife/husband]**, _____, and in the proportions they would so inherit under the laws of the State of _____ as though **[she/he]** had died intestate and domiciled in the State of _____ at the time distribution is so to be made.

C. If the Trustee is authorized pursuant to the provisions of this Article III to make distributions or payments to or for the benefit of any person (including distributions or payments directed or permitted to be made to a person who is under legal disability or, in the reasonable opinion of the Trustee, is unable properly to administer such distributions or payments), the Trustee may make such distributions or payments in any one or more of the following ways, as the Trustee may deem advisable: (1) directly to such beneficiary; (2) to the legal guardian of such beneficiary; (3) to any custodian then serving for such beneficiary, or to any person designated by the Trustee to serve as a custodian for such beneficiary (any such custodian may be the Trustee); or (4) by the Trustee itself expending such income or principal for the benefit of such beneficiary. The Trustee shall not be required to see to the application of any distribution or payment so made, but the receipt of any of the persons mentioned in Clause (1), (2) or (3) in the immediately preceding sentence shall be a full discharge for the Trustee.

D. All interests of a beneficiary hereunder shall be inalienable and free from anticipation, assignment, attachment, pledge or control by creditors or a present or former spouse of such beneficiary in any proceedings at law or in equity.

E. Any provisions of this Article III to the contrary notwithstanding, if not already distributed, all accrued and undistributed income and the entire principal of every trust estate then held hereunder shall be paid over and distributed outright and free of the trust not later than the end of the day immediately preceding the expiration of twenty-one (21) years from and after the death of the last survivor of myself, my children and my children's issue living at the time of my death. Such payment and distribution shall be made to the person or persons for whose benefit the trust estate or estates respectively shall then be held hereunder.

ARTICLE IV

DEFINITIONS

A. The words "issue," "child" and "children," as used herein, shall be deemed to include any legally adopted person as if he or she were the natural child of the adopting parent.

B. Whenever the context so requires, the use of words herein in the singular shall be construed to include the plural, and words in the plural, the singular, and words whether in the masculine, feminine or neuter gender shall be construed to include all of said genders.

ARTICLE V

POWERS AND DUTIES OF THE TRUSTEE

A. There shall be no duty on the Trustee to pay or see to the payment of any premiums on any policies of life insurance or to take any steps to keep them in force, until such time as the

Trustee holds title to any insurance policies hereunder as a part of the corpus of any trust estate. The Trustee furthermore assumes no responsibility with respect to the validity or enforceability of said policies. However, as soon as practicable after receiving notice of the death of the insured under any of such policies, the Trustee shall proceed to collect all amounts payable thereunder. The Trustee shall have full and complete authority to collect and receive any and all such amounts and its receipt therefor shall be a full and complete acquittance to any insurer or payor, who shall be under no obligation to see to the proper application thereof by the Trustee.

B. In the administration of the trusts created hereunder and in addition to the powers exercised by trustees generally, the Trustee shall have the following powers and authorities without any court order or proceeding, exercisable in the discretion of the Trustee:

1. To purchase as an investment for the trust estate or estates any property, real or personal, belonging to my estate;

2. To retain as suitable investments for the trust estate or estates any properties (including, without limitation, securities issued by any corporate Trustee or the holding company of which it is an affiliate) received by it from me, and/or my estate, and whether received by purchase or in any other manner, without regard to any law, statutory or judicial, or any rule or practice of court now or hereafter in force specifying or limiting the permissible investments of trustees, trust companies or fiduciaries generally or requiring the diversification of investments, and without liability to any person whomsoever for loss or depreciation in value thereof;

3. To sell, exchange, convey, mortgage, pledge, lease, control, and manage, and to make contracts concerning, any of the properties, real or personal, comprised in the trust estate or estates, all either publicly or privately and for such considerations and upon such terms as to credit or otherwise as may be reasonable under the circumstances, which leases and contracts may extend beyond the duration of any of the trusts created hereunder; to give options therefor; and to execute deeds, transfers, mortgages, leases and other instruments of any kind;

4. To invest and reinvest the properties from time to time comprised in the trust estate or estates in stocks, common and/or preferred, bonds, notes, debentures, loans, mortgages, common trust funds, or other securities or property, real or personal, all limitations now or hereafter imposed by law, statutory or judicial, or by any rule or practice of court now or hereafter in force specifying or limiting the permissible investments of trustees, trust companies or fiduciaries generally or requiring the diversification of investments, being hereby expressly waived, it being the intent hereof that the Trustee shall have full power and authority to deal with the trust estate or estates in all respects as though it was the sole owner thereof, without order of court or other authority;

5. To borrow money, from itself or otherwise, with or without security, whenever it deems such action advisable;

6. To exercise voting rights, execute and deliver powers of attorney and proxies and similarly act with reference to shares of stock and other securities comprised in the trust estate or estates in such manner as it deems proper, including, without limitation, the power to participate in or oppose reorganizations, recapitalizations, mergers, consolidations, exchanges, liquidations, arrangements and other corporate actions;

7. To collect all money; in accordance with generally accepted trust accounting principles, to determine whether money or other property coming into its possession shall be treated as principal or income and to charge or apportion expenses, taxes, gains and losses to principal or income;

8. To compromise, adjust and settle claims in favor of or against the trust estate or estates upon such terms and conditions as it may deem best; in the case of any

3

litigation in connection with any part of such trust estate or estates, it may, under advice of its counsel, arbitrate, settle, or adjust any such matter in dispute upon such terms as it may consider just and equitable, and its decision shall be binding upon the beneficiaries;

9. To employ investment counsel, custodians of estate property, brokers, accountants, attorneys, clerical or bookkeeping assistants, and other suitable agents and to pay their reasonable compensation and expenses in addition to any compensation payable to the Trustee, and to execute and deliver powers of attorney; the Trustee shall not be liable for any neglect, omission or wrongdoing of such investment counsel, custodians, brokers, accountants, attorneys, assistants or agents, provided reasonable care shall have been exercised in their selection;

10. To hold title to stocks, bonds, or other securities or property, real or personal, in its own name or in the name of its nominee and without indication of any fiduciary capacity or to hold any such bonds or securities in bearer form; the Trustee shall assume full responsibility for the acts of any nominee selected by it;

11. To make all repairs, alterations or improvements of any real property which shall constitute a part of the trust estate or estates; adjust boundaries thereof, and to erect or demolish buildings thereon; and, with respect to such property, to convert for different use, grant easements for adequate consideration, partition, and insure for any or all risks;

12. To pay premiums on any policies of life insurance which may form a part of the trust estate or estates; to cancel, sell, assign, hypothecate, pledge or otherwise dispose of any of said policies; to exercise any right, election, option or privilege granted by any of said policies; to borrow any sums in accordance with the provisions of any of said policies, and to receive all payments, dividends, surrender values, additions, benefits or privileges of any kind which may accrue to any of said policies;

13. To make any allocation, division or distribution required or permitted hereunder in cash or in kind, in real or personal property, or an undivided interest therein, or partly in cash and partly in kind, and to do so without making pro rata allocations, divisions or distributions of specific assets, property allocated, divided or distributed in kind to be taken at its fair market value at the time of such allocation, division or distribution;

14. To receive, in accordance with the provisions of Article I hereof, additional property from me or any other person, the Trustee being authorized and empowered to merge and hold as one any duplicate trusts held for the same beneficiary;

15. To make such expenditures and do such other acts as are reasonably required to manage, improve, protect, preserve, invest or sell any of the trust estates or otherwise properly to administer this Trust.

C. If the representative of my estate, in such representative's sole discretion, shall determine that appropriate assets of my estate are not available in sufficient amount to pay (a) taxes levied against or with respect to my taxable estate by reason of my death, including interest and penalties thereon, if any, and (b) expenses of administration of my estate, the Trustee shall, upon the request of the representative of my estate, contribute from the principal of the trust estate the amount of such deficiency; and in connection with any such action the Trustee shall rely upon the written statement of the representative of my estate as to the validity and correctness of the amounts of any such taxes, expenses and bequests, and shall furnish funds to such representative so as to enable such representative to discharge the same, or to discharge any part or all thereof themselves by making payment directly to the governmental official or agency or to the person entitled or claiming to be entitled to receive payment thereof. No consideration need be required by the Trustee from the representative of my estate for any disbursement made by the Trustee pursuant hereto, nor shall there be any obligation upon such representative to repay to the Trustee any of the funds disbursed by it hereunder, and all amounts disbursed by the Trustee pursuant to the authority hereby conferred upon it shall be disbursed without any right in or duty upon the Trustee to seek or obtain contribution or reimbursement from any person or property on account of such payment. The Trustee shall not be responsible for the application of any funds delivered by it to the representative of my estate pursuant to the authority herein granted, nor shall the Trustee be subject to liability to any beneficiary hereunder on account of any payment made by it pursuant to the provisions hereof.

    D. The Trustee shall keep accurate records showing all receipts and disbursements and other transactions involving the trust estate or estates and shall furnish annually to each beneficiary currently entitled to income, (1) a statement of the receipts and disbursements affecting such beneficiary's interest in the trust, and (2) a complete inventory of the trust estate then held for the benefit of such beneficiary.

    E. No person, firm or corporation dealing with the Trustee or a nominee of the Trustee or performing any act pursuant to action taken or order given by the Trustee or such nominee shall be obliged to inquire as to the propriety, validity or legality thereof hereunder, nor shall any such person be liable for the application of any money or other consideration paid to the Trustee or such nominee, but, instead, may rely upon any action taken by the Trustee or such nominee pursuant to the powers and authorities conferred upon it under the provisions of this Article V in all respects as if the same were completely unlimited. No transfer agent or registrar of any security held hereunder shall be required to inquire as to the propriety, validity or legality of any transfer made by the Trustee or such nominee.

    F. 1. In the event that said _____ shall be unwilling or unable to continue to serve as Trustee hereunder, then, my _____, _____, of _____, _____, shall serve as successor Trustee hereunder. In the event that both said _____ and said _____ shall be unwilling or unable to serve or continue to serve as Trustee hereunder, then _____, of _____, _____, shall serve as successor Trustee hereunder. Any Trustee shall be entitled to resign as Trustee for any reason whatsoever by giving written notice to the Trustee designated to succeed it; provided that the Trustee designated to succeed it shall first execute a formal written acceptance of the duties and obligations of the Trustee hereunder and file an executed copy of such acceptance with the preceding Trustee. After this is done, and when all sums then due from the trust estate to such predecessor Trustee have been paid, such predecessor Trustee shall transfer the Trust property then in its hands to such successor Trustee and such predecessor Trustee shall thereupon and thereby be discharged of all subsequent duties and obligations under or arising out of its trusteeship.

    2. Any successor Trustee shall have and enjoy all the powers, authorities, duties and immunities hereby vested in and imposed upon the original Trustee and no successor Trustee shall be obliged to inquire into or be in any way accountable for the previous administration of the trust property.

    G. My Trustee is authorized, in its discretion, to sell to, purchase from, borrow funds from, lend funds to, or otherwise deal with, upon such terms and conditions as my Trustee shall deem just and equitable and for full and adequate consideration, the Executor of the Last Will and Testament of myself or the Trustee of any Trust established by me (whether such Trust is a testamentary or inter vivos trust), even though my Trustee may also be serving as Executor under my Will or as Trustee under any such Trust established by me.

    H. In determining the amount of any discretionary distributions of income or principal to a beneficiary of a trust created hereunder, the Trustee shall be required to take into account all other means and resources known to or reasonably ascertainable by the Trustee, including Medicaid or any other form of government assistance, which are available to such beneficiary for the purposes for which the Trustee is authorized to make said distributions.

I. _____, as Trustee, shall serve without compensation. Any other Trustee shall be entitled to receive reasonable compensation. Any Trustee shall be entitled to be reimbursed for reasonable expenses it incurs which are necessary to carry out its duties as Trustee hereunder.

J. No bond shall be required of the Trustee hereunder or any successor Trustee.

K. The Trustee and any successor Trustee are specifically instructed by the Settlor to maintain the privacy and confidentiality of this instrument and the trust created hereunder, and are in no circumstances to divulge its terms to any probate or other court or other public agency with the exception of a tax authority.

L. The Trustee and any successor Trustee shall have the authority to merge any trust held hereunder with any other trust, however created, which has similar provisions, the same beneficiaries and the same Trustee.

M. Notwithstanding any other provision contained herein, an individual Trustee (a) shall have no incident of ownership or power with respect to any policy of insurance upon such Trustee's life, and (b) shall have no power or discretion with respect to the allocation or distribution of assets to the extent that such would discharge such Trustee's legal obligation to support any beneficiary, or directly or indirectly benefit such Trustee unless necessary to provide for such Trustee's support in reasonable comfort, health care or education at any level, considering such Trustee's other financial resources.

ARTICLE VI

GOVERNING LAW

This Trust Agreement shall be construed under and in accordance with the laws of the State of _____.

IN WITNESS WHEREOF, I have hereunto set my hand, and the Trustee, to evidence its acceptance of the Trust herein expressed, has hereunto set its hand, in duplicate, at _____ _____, _____, on the day and year first above written.

Signed in the presence of:

_____   _____

_____   _____
                                                                  "Settlor"

_____   _____

_____   _____
                                                                  "Trustee"

STATE OF _____   City
                                          or
COUNTY OF _____   Town _____

On the _____ day of _____, 19____, personally appeared _____ known to me to be the individual(s) who executed the foregoing instrument, and acknowledged the same to be **[his/her]** free act and deed, before me.

My commission expires: _____
                                          Notary Public

_____

6

SCHEDULE A

The following is a true and correct Schedule A of the property assigned, delivered and conveyed to _____, Trustee, to be held, treated and disposed of in accordance with the terms of a certain Irrevocable Trust Agreement between _____, the Settlor, and _____, the Trustee, dated _____ ____, 19____, to which Agreement this Schedule A is attached and made a part thereof.

_____

_____

_____

_____

_____

_____

_____

_____

_____

_____

_____

_____

_____

_____

_____

_____

_____

_____

_____

_____

Signed in the presence of:

_____   _____

_____   _____
                                                                   "Settlor"

_____   _____

_____   _____
                                                                   "Trustee"

ADDITION OF PROPERTY TO IRREVOCABLE TRUST AGREEMENT

BY _____

DATED _____ ___, 19___

WITH _____, TRUSTEE

_____ (the "Assignor"), pursuant to the terms of the above-described Irrevocable Trust Agreement, does hereby assign, transfer and convey to _____,

Trustee, and _____,

Trustee, does hereby acknowledge receipt of, the following assets from the Assignor:

_____

_____

_____

_____

_____

_____

_____

_____

_____

_____

_____

_____

_____

_____

_____

_____

The Trustee agrees to hold, manage and administer the above assets as a part of the trust estate created under such Irrevocable Trust Agreement.

At the request of the Trustee, the Assignor shall fully cooperate and execute any and all documents deemed necessary or desirable by it in order to cause the assignment made hereby to be properly recorded.

IN WITNESS WHEREOF, the Assignor and the Trustee have signed their names at _____, _____, on this ____ day of _____, 19___.

Signed in the presence of:

_____   _____

_____   _____, Assignor

_____   _____

_____   _____, Trustee

8

STATE OF _____   City
                                     or
COUNTY OF _____   Town _____

      On the _____ day of _____, 19____, personally appeared
_____ known to me to be the individual(s) who executed the fore-
going instrument, and acknowledged the same to be **[his/her]** free act and deed, before me.

                                                             _____
                                                             Notary Public

My commission expires:
_____

Medicaid Trust No. 4
for Individual Who Is Unmarried, Leaving Assets Equally to Children

Instructions/Explanation

As you can readily see, the trust agreement is filled with legalese. Don't be scared off by this confusing language. The explanations that follow should provide you with a clear understanding of the terms used.

Introduction: In the first blanks, fill in the city and state where you reside and the day, month, and year in which you are executing the Agreement.

Next, put in your name and residence (city and state)—the "Settlor" is your title when you make a trust. Then fill in the name, city, and state of the person or institution whom you are naming as trustee.

Remember, you should not be the trustee. A child or other close relative will probably be your first choice (keeping in mind possible tax consequences where annual distributions of over $10,000 will be made). If no one fits that description, you may have to name an institutional trustee, such as a bank.

Article I(A): This is the section making your trust irrevocable. Once you sign the Agreement, you will never be able to change, amend, or revoke it.

Article I(B): This paragraph transfers into the Trust all the items listed on Schedule A at the end of the Agreement. You can include on Schedule A just about any item imaginable, including real estate, personal property, savings and checking accounts, boats, cars, even clothing.

If the property you put into the trust increases in value, the increased value is part of the trust. And if an asset changes form, the new asset still remains in the trust. For example, if the trustee takes $5,000 from a bank account and buys $5,000 worth of stock, the stock remains in the trust.

While you can never remove assets once they are placed into the trust, you can always add to the trust by using the Addition to Trust form following Schedule A.

A testamentary gift, referred to in this paragraph, is a gift given at the time of someone's death, normally contained in a will. For example, you may not put your car into trust immediately, but you may add to your trust under your will when you die.

Article II: This section gives you the income from the trust during your life, but specifically provides that you cannot get at the principal. This is *absolutely crucial* to saving your estate from the grasp of a nursing home if you enter one. With this language, Medicaid cannot require you to spend the principal on the nursing home *because you don't control or even have access to the principal.*

Why does the Trust Agreement give discretion to the Trustee to pay you income rather than *requiring* the Trustee to pay you all the income? Because with this provision, you *may* be able to protect your income from the nursing home.

Let's say the Trust Agreement just said that all the income was automatically yours. If you entered a nursing home, Medicaid would force you to pay all the income to the nursing home and would only cover any deficiency on the bill. But if the Trustee has discretion to decide whether or not to pay all the income to you, after you go into a nursing home the Trustee might decide *not* to pay *any* of the income to you. In that situation, Medicaid might pay the entire nursing-home tab, because you don't have any income. (I say might because the law and its application to situations like this are not yet clear. It is possible that Medicaid might say that, even if you're not actually receiving any income, you *could* receive some or all of the income and so it won't pay the full nursing-home bill.)

Article III: This section describes how your trust principal, less any of your estate taxes, estate administration costs, or funeral expenses as provided in Article V(C) will be distributed after you die.

Paragraph III(A) provides that, after you die, the balance of your trust principal will be distributed equally to your children. If any of your children has died before you, that child's portion goes to that child's children.

Paragraph III(B) provides for the distribution of the trust if there's no one to receive the principal from your trust under Paragraph III(A). If you die leaving no living children or grandchildren, Paragraph III(B) takes over.

Under III(B), the remaining principal of the trust will be divided into two parts. One part will go to those persons who would inherit from you under the laws of your state as if you had died without a will or a trust. Every state has a law that dictates to whom an estate of someone who dies without a will will be distributed—usually to the closest living relative(s) of the deceased. For example, if you die without children or grandchildren, Paragraph III(B) may mean that your parent or brother collects part of the trust estate.

The other half of the trust estate will be distributed to those persons who would inherit from your deceased spouse under the laws of your state as if he or she had died without a will.

The estate is split into two parts so that relatives on both sides of your family are treated equally. For example, rather than having everything go to your cousin, half may go to your cousin and half to your deceased spouse's sister.

Fill in the blanks in Paragraph III(B) with the names of your state and your deceased spouse (if any).

Part III(C) discusses distributions, after you die, to beneficiaries named in your trust who are under some legal disability or are unable to administer their distributions. For example, if your child is senile or suffering from Alzheimer's disease, he or she may be under a legal disability or unable to manage his or her money. Or if a distribution under your trust is to go to a young child (perhaps the children of a deceased child of yours), Part III(C) may come into play.

If a distribution from your trust is to go to someone who is under a legal disability or unable to manage their money, the Trustee has four options:

1. Pay the money to the beneficiary.
2. Make the distribution to a legal guardian of the beneficiary.
3. Distribute the beneficiary's portion to a custodian for the beneficiary.
4. Spend the money himself or herself for the benefit of the beneficiary.

If, when you make up your trust, you could predict the ages and physical and mental conditions of all your beneficiaries at the time of your death, you could spell out which of these four options you would want the Trustee to pursue. But since you can't, this Trust allows the Trustee to choose which option he or she believes is best.

The last sentence of Part III(C) says that, once the Trustee has made his or her choice and distributed a beneficiary's portion to the beneficiary or to the beneficiary's guardian or custodian, the Trustee is off the hook; he or she doesn't have to monitor the use of the distribution after that.

Part III(D), often called a spendthrift clause, provides that nobody but your intended beneficiary can obtain an interest in a distribution under your Trust. For example, your child, who will receive a portion of your Trust after you're gone, can't sell his or her expected distribution in the future to someone for cash now. And a beneficiary can't put up his or her interest in a distribution as collateral for a loan. After all, you want the person you name in the Trust to receive a distribution, not some stranger.

Spendthrift clauses like this are enforced in most, but not all, states. If you have a serious concern that a beneficiary has or may have creditor problems, consult with a local attorney to determine whether this clause will be effective in your state.

Trusts cannot legally tie up assets forever, so Part III(E) is designed to avoid potential problems by limiting the life of the Trust.

Article IV: This is the definition section. The only important point here is to recognize that a legally adopted child will be considered a child for purposes of the Trust Agreement. So by leaving everything to your children equally after you die, any adopted child would be treated the same as a natural child.

Article V: This section deals with the powers and duties you are giving to the Trustee.

Part V(A) says that, after your death, the Trustee must collect the money due under any insurance policy on your life. The Trustee does not have a duty to pay your life insurance premiums during your lifetime, until and unless the Trustee takes title to any insurance policy.

Part V(B) is very important, setting forth the powers of the Trustee. As you can see, this Trust Agreement gives the Trustee very broad powers to administer the funds and property in the estate, including the power to:

1. Buy real estate or personal property from your estate. Without this power, purchases

2. Keep in the Trust anything received from you or your estate.

3. Sell, exchange, mortgage, and do just about anything else with property in the Trust.

4. Invest the assets in the Trust in just about anything.

5. Borrow money for the Trust.

6. Manage stock and other securities.

7. Collect money for the Trust.

8. Handle claims and lawsuits for or against the Trust.

9. Hire and pay counselors and assistants, like lawyers and accountants, for the Trust.

10. Hold property in his or her own name, in the name of a nominee, or in bearer form.

11. Manage real estate in the Trust, including repairing, improving, or converting property.

12. Handle life insurance policies in the Trust, including paying premiums, canceling or selling policies, cashing in policies, or borrowing against them.

13. Make distributions under the Trust in cash or in property.

14. Receive additional property for the Trust.

15. Do anything else reasonably required to manage, protect, or preserve the Trust assets.

Why put in many specific powers, instead of just having item 15, which generally allows the Trustee to do anything reasonably necessary? Because with only a general statement, someone with whom the Trustee must deal may question his or her power and may refuse to do business with him or her. For example, without specifically giving the Trustee the power to sell real estate, buyers, lenders, and escrow agents may be hesitant to deal with him or her, even if your trust agreement generally gives him or her broad powers. By listing specific powers, you can ensure the Trustee's ability properly to manage the Trust.

Why give the Trustee such broad powers anyway? Why not just specify a few actions he or she may take? The reason is simple: you can't predict what the Trustee may need to do to manage your estate properly, and if you don't give him or her broad powers, you may hamper him or her and damage your Trust estate. For example, if you don't own any stocks, why give the Trustee power to manage them? Because at some point it might be in your

by your Trustee from your estate at death might not be allowed.

best interest for your Trustee to purchase securities, and your Trust Agreement could unnecessarily prevent him or her from doing so.

Part V(C) provides for certain payments from your Trust upon your death. If the representative of your estate (such as the executor or administrator) decides that the funds left in your estate (not in your Trust) are insufficient to pay your estate taxes, expenses of administration, or funeral expenses, he or she can require the Trustee to cover those costs. The Trustee does not have to get anything in return, and your estate representative does not have to repay the money. Once the Trustee has paid the representative of your estate, the Trustee has no further obligation to monitor the use of these funds.

Part V(D) requires the Trustee to keep accurate records showing all transactions in the Trust. Every year, the Trustee must give to certain beneficiaries a statement listing the Trust transactions for the year and a current inventory of assets in the Trust. Not every possible future beneficiary of the Trust gets this report. For example, if the Trust Agreement provides income to you for your lifetime, then on your death the assets will be distributed to your children or their children, only you are entitled to the Trustee's report.

Part V(E) is designed to encourage people to deal with the Trustee by relieving them of liability in case the Trustee takes some action beyond his power. For example, if the Trustee attempts to sell a house, the buyer can go ahead with the transaction and pay the Trustee without worrying about whether the Trust really allows the Trustee to make that deal.

Part V(F)(1) allows you to name alternative Trustees in case your first and/or second choice can't or won't serve when the time comes. In the first blank, put the name of your first choice for Trustee. In the next three blanks, fill in the relationship to you, the name and residence of your second choice. In the next two blanks, fill in the names of your first and second choices for Trustee. In the last three blanks, include the name, city, and state of a third choice for Trustee.

Part V(F)(2) gives any successor Trustee all the same powers and duties as the original Trustee. It also encourages your chosen successor Trustee to accept the job by providing that he or she has no responsibility for anything done by the earlier Trustee.

Part V(G) authorizes the Trustee to engage in

transactions with the Executor of your estate or any trustee of any other trust established by you. Without this language, a conflict-of-interest issue could arise over these types of dealings.

Part V(H) concerns discretionary distributions by the Trustee. Under Article II, the Trustee is given discretion to distribute to you all the net income of the trust. Let's say you enter a nursing home—will some or all of the income from the trust have to be paid to the nursing home? Under the law as it stands now, the answer is not totally clear. Medicaid may take the position that *all* the income must be paid to you (and so to the nursing home). But with Part V(H), there is a chance you can save part or all of the income.

Under Part V(H), the Trustee could decide not to pay any of the income to you. In fact, by requiring the Trustee to consider other resources available, including Medicaid, you are tilting the Trustee's decision in the direction of nonpayment. If the Trustee makes that decision, Medicaid might allow the trust to retain the income while it pays your nursing-home costs.

In Part V(I), you are providing that the Trustee (whose name must be filled in the blank) will serve without compensation. Since the Trustee will probably be your child or someone else close to you, that should be agreeable. Other possible trustees, such as a bank, will want to be paid, and Part V(I) allows that as well.

Part V(J) states that the Trustee does not have to post a bond. A bond is like an insurance policy, designed to protect your Trust in case the Trustee does something wrong, such as steals assets. Depending on the amount in the Trust, the bond could easily cost your Trust several hundred dollars. If you've followed the tips in this book and selected the right Trustee, you shouldn't need a bond.

Part V(K) instructs the Trustee to keep the terms of your Trust private to the maximum extent possible. A trust has a great advantage over a will when it comes to passing your assets along after your death. Your estate becomes an open book when it goes through probate; when it passes under a trust, it can be kept from the eyes of nosy neighbors.

Part V(L) allows the Trustee to merge trusts that are very similar to avoid duplication of effort and costs.

Part V(M) is a protection for the Trustee to avoid the remote possibility of having the trust property included in the Trustee's estate, causing adverse tax consequences.

Article VI: Article VI states that any questions about the Trust will be answered by the laws of the state of your primary residence. In the blank space, fill in the name of your state.

Conclusion: In the blanks in the final paragraph, fill in your city and state. Then sign where it says Settlor (that's you) and have the Trustee sign below that. You and the Trustee should each print your names below the signature lines. To the left of your and the Trustee's signatures, two witnesses to each signature must sign. The witnesses can be the same, but they don't have to be; if they are the same, they must sign twice (once for the Settlor and once for the Trustee). The witnesses cannot be members of your family.

The final section is for a notary public.

Schedule A: Following the end of the Trust is Schedule A, on which you should list any items (i.e., cash accounts, real estate, personal property, etc.) to be placed under the control of the Trustee. Identify each item as best you can, using addresses, registration numbers, account numbers, etc., wherever possible, to avoid confusion.

On Schedule A, fill in: the name of the Trustee in the first blank, your name (the "Settlor") in the second blank, and the name of the Trustee again in the third blank. Then date the Schedule.

At the bottom, you and the Trustee should sign before two independent witnesses.

Addition of Property Form: Finally included is a form that you can use to add property to the Trust later. At the top, fill in your name, the date that the Trust was originally made, and the name of the Trustee. In the first full paragraph, fill in your name as the Assignor, assigning property to the Trustee. Then on the lines that follow, list any items to be added to the Trust. Again, identify each item as best you can. At the end, you and the Trustee should sign before two independent witnesses and a notary.

IRREVOCABLE TRUST AGREEMENT

THIS IRREVOCABLE TRUST AGREEMENT is entered into at _____
_____, _____, this _____ day of _____, 19___, by and
between _____, of _____,
_____, the Settlor, hereinafter referred to in the first person,
and _____, of _____,
_____, the Trustee, hereinafter referred to as the "Trustee" and
sometimes in the third person impersonal.

ARTICLE I

CREATION OF TRUST

A. Except as provided in Paragraph B of this Article I, this Trust Agreement shall be
irrevocable, and I hereby expressly acknowledge that I shall have no right or power, either alone or
in conjunction with others, and in any capacity whatsoever, to alter, amend, modify, revoke or terminate
this Trust or any of the terms of this Trust Agreement in whole or in part, or otherwise to cause any
of the assets of the Trust to revert to me or to my estate.

B. I hereby transfer the property listed in Schedule A of this Trust Agreement to the
Trustee. That property and all proceeds, investments and reinvestments thereof and any property
hereinafter received by the Trustee from me, or from any other person (such property being hereinafter referred to as the "trust estate"), shall be held, administered and distributed in accordance with
the terms of the trust herein expressed. I reserve to myself and to others the right to add property to
the trust estate by lifetime or testamentary gifts, all of which added property shall be governed by the
terms hereof.

ARTICLE II

DISTRIBUTIONS DURING LIFETIME OF SETTLOR

During my lifetime, the Trustee may distribute to or for the benefit of me, out of the net
income of the trust estate, such amount or amounts as the Trustee deems necessary to provide for my
maintenance and support. At the end of each taxable year the Trustee shall add any undistributed
income to the principal of the trust estate being held hereunder.

ARTICLE III

DIVISION OF TRUST ESTATE UPON SETTLOR'S DEATH

Upon my death, the Trustee shall hold, administer and distribute the property held
hereunder, as the same shall be constituted after being (a) augmented by property received or to be
received by the Trustee as a consequence of my death, including, without limitation, any property
received or to be received under the terms of my Last Will and Testament or any Codicil thereto and
(b) depleted by any money disbursed by the Trustee pursuant to the provisions of Paragraph C of
Article V hereof (said property as so constituted being hereinafter referred to as "The Family Trust")
in accordance with the following provisions of this Trust Agreement.

A. Upon my death, the Trustee shall distribute the balance of The Family Trust being
held hereunder to the following persons who survive me in the proportions shown, treating as a surviving
person the then living collective issue of any such person who shall then be deceased, the distribution
to such issue to be *per stirpes*, the root of the *per stirpes* distribution to be such predeceased person.

Name	Proportion To Be Paid
_____	_____%
_____	_____%
_____	_____%
_____	_____%
_____	_____%
_____	_____%

B. If at the time for distribution of The Family Trust or any share or portion of the trust estate being held pursuant to this Article III, there is no person or person's estate entitled under the provisions of this Article III other than this Paragraph B to take such distribution, the Trustee shall divide the trust estate into two (2) equal shares. One such share shall be distributed free of the trust to such person or persons as would be entitled to inherit from me and in the proportions they would so inherit under the laws of the State of _____ as though I had died intestate and domiciled in the State of _____ at the time distribution is so to be made. The other such share shall be distributed free of the trust to such person or persons as would be entitled to inherit from my deceased **[wife/husband]**, _____, and in the proportions they would so inherit under the laws of the State of _____ as though **[he/she]** had died intestate and domiciled in the State of _____ at the time distribution is so to be made.

C. If the Trustee is authorized pursuant to the provisions of this Article III to make distributions or payments to or for the benefit of any person (including distributions or payments directed or permitted to be made to a person who is under legal disability or, in the reasonable opinion of the Trustee, is unable properly to administer such distributions or payments), the Trustee may make such distributions or payments in any one or more of the following ways, as the Trustee may deem advisable: (1) directly to such beneficiary; (2) to the legal guardian of such beneficiary; (3) to any custodian then serving for such beneficiary, or to any person designated by the Trustee to serve as a custodian for such beneficiary (any such custodian may be the Trustee); or (4) by the Trustee itself expending such income or principal for the benefit of such beneficiary. The Trustee shall not be required to see to the application of any distribution or payment so made, but the receipt of any of the persons mentioned in Clause (1), (2) or (3) in the immediately preceding sentence shall be a full discharge for the Trustee.

D. All interests of a beneficiary hereunder shall be inalienable and free from anticipation, assignment, attachment, pledge or control by creditors or a present or former spouse of such beneficiary in any proceedings at law or in equity.

E. Any provisions of this Article III to the contrary notwithstanding, if not already distributed, all accrued and undistributed income and the entire principal of every trust estate then held hereunder shall be paid over and distributed outright and free of the trust not later than the end of the day immediately preceding the expiration of twenty-one (21) years from and after the death of the last survivor of myself, my children and my children's issue living at the time of my death. Such payment and distribution shall be made to the person or persons for whose benefit the trust estate or estates respectively shall then be held hereunder.

ARTICLE IV

DEFINITIONS

A. The words "issue," "child" and "children," as used herein, shall be deemed to include any legally adopted person as if he or she were the natural child of the adopting parent.

B. Whenever the context so requires, the use of words herein in the singular shall be construed to include the plural, and words in the plural, the singular, and words whether in the masculine, feminine or neuter gender shall be construed to include all of said genders.

ARTICLE V

POWERS AND DUTIES OF THE TRUSTEE

A. There shall be no duty on the Trustee to pay or see to the payment of any premiums on any policies of life insurance or to take any steps to keep them in force, until such time as the Trustee holds title to any insurance policies hereunder as a part of the corpus of any trust estate. The Trustee furthermore assumes no responsibility with respect to the validity or enforceability of said policies. However, as soon as practicable after receiving notice of the death of the insured under any of such policies, the Trustee shall proceed to collect all amounts payable thereunder. The Trustee shall have full and complete authority to collect and receive any and all such amounts and its receipt therefor shall be a full and complete acquittance to any insurer or payor, who shall be under no obligation to see to the proper application thereof by the Trustee.

B. In the administration of the trusts created hereunder and in addition to the powers exercised by trustees generally, the Trustee shall have the following powers and authorities without any court order or proceeding, exercisable in the discretion of the Trustee:

1. To purchase as an investment for the trust estate or estates any property, real or personal, belonging to my estate;

2. To retain as suitable investments for the trust estate or estates any properties (including, without limitation, securities issued by any corporate Trustee or the holding company of which it is an affiliate) received by it from me, and/or my estate, and whether received by purchase or in any other manner, without regard to any law, statutory or judicial, or any rule or practice of court now or hereafter in force specifying or limiting the permissible investments of trustees, trust companies or fiduciaries generally or requiring the diversification of investments, and without liability to any person whomsoever for loss or depreciation in value thereof;

3. To sell, exchange, convey, mortgage, pledge, lease, control, and manage, and to make contracts concerning, any of the properties, real or personal, comprised in the trust estate or estates, all either publicly or privately and for such considerations and upon such terms as to credit or otherwise as may be reasonable under the circumstances, which leases and contracts may extend beyond the duration of any of the trusts created hereunder; to give options therefor; and to execute deeds, transfers, mortgages, leases and other instruments of any kind;

4. To invest and reinvest the properties from time to time comprised in the trust estate or estates in stocks, common and/or preferred, bonds, notes, debentures, loans, mortgages, common trust funds, or other securities or property, real or personal, all limitations now or hereafter imposed by law, statutory or judicial, or by any rule or practice of court now or hereafter in force specifying or limiting the permissible investments of trustees, trust companies or fiduciaries generally or requiring the diversification of investments, being hereby expressly waived, it being the intent hereof that the Trustee shall have full power and authority to deal with the trust estate or estates in all respects as though it was the sole owner thereof, without order of court or other authority;

5. To borrow money, from itself or otherwise, with or without security, whenever it deems such action advisable;

6. To exercise voting rights, execute and deliver powers of attorney and proxies and similarly act with reference to shares of stock and other securities comprised in the trust estate or estates in such manner as it deems proper, including, without

limitation, the power to participate in or oppose reorganizations, recapitalizations, mergers, consolidations, exchanges, liquidations, arrangements and other corporate actions;

7. To collect all money; in accordance with generally accepted trust accounting principles, to determine whether money or other property coming into its possession shall be treated as principal or income and to charge or apportion expenses, taxes, gains and losses to principal or income;

8. To compromise, adjust and settle claims in favor of or against the trust estate or estates upon such terms and conditions as it may deem best; in the case of any litigation in connection with any part of such trust estate or estates, it may, under advice of its counsel, arbitrate, settle, or adjust any such matter in dispute upon such terms as it may consider just and equitable, and its decision shall be binding upon the beneficiaries;

9. To employ investment counsel, custodians of estate property, brokers, accountants, attorneys, clerical or bookkeeping assistants, and other suitable agents and to pay their reasonable compensation and expenses in addition to any compensation payable to the Trustee, and to execute and deliver powers of attorney; the Trustee shall not be liable for any neglect, omission or wrongdoing of such investment counsel, custodians, brokers, accountants, attorneys, assistants or agents, provided reasonable care shall have been exercised in their selection;

10. To hold title to stocks, bonds, or other securities or property, real or personal, in its own name or in the name of its nominee and without indication of any fiduciary capacity or to hold any such bonds or securities in bearer form; the Trustee shall assume full responsibility for the acts of any nominee selected by it;

11. To make all repairs, alterations or improvements of any real property which shall constitute a part of the trust estate or estates; adjust boundaries thereof, and to erect or demolish buildings thereon; and, with respect to such property, to convert for different use, grant easements for adequate consideration, partition, and insure for any or all risks;

12. To pay premiums on any policies of life insurance which may form a part of the trust estate or estates; to cancel, sell, assign, hypothecate, pledge or otherwise dispose of any of said policies; to exercise any right, election, option or privilege granted by any of said policies; to borrow any sums in accordance with the provisions of any of said policies, and to receive all payments, dividends, surrender values, additions, benefits or privileges of any kind which may accrue to any of said policies;

13. To make any allocation, division or distribution required or permitted hereunder in cash or in kind, in real or personal property, or an undivided interest therein, or partly in cash and partly in kind, and to do so without making pro rata allocations, divisions or distributions of specific assets, property allocated, divided or distributed in kind to be taken at its fair market value at the time of such allocation, division or distribution;

14. To receive, in accordance with the provisions of Article I hereof, additional property from me or any other person, the Trustee being authorized and empowered to merge and hold as one any duplicate trusts held for the same beneficiary;

15. To make such expenditures and do such other acts as are reasonably required to manage, improve, protect, preserve, invest or sell any of the trust estates or otherwise properly to administer this Trust.

C. If the representative of my estate, in such representative's sole discretion, shall determine that appropriate assets of my estate are not available in sufficient amount to pay (a) taxes levied against or with respect to my taxable estate by reason of my death, including interest and penalties thereon, if any, and (b) expenses of administration of my estate, the Trustee shall, upon the request of the representative of my estate, contribute from the principal of the trust estate the amount of such deficiency; and in connection with any such action the Trustee shall rely upon the written statement of the representative of my estate as to the validity and correctness of the amounts of any such taxes, expenses and bequests, and shall furnish funds to such representative so as to enable such representative to discharge the same, or to discharge any part or all thereof themselves by making payment directly to the governmental official or agency or to the person entitled or claiming to be entitled to receive payment thereof. No consideration need be required by the Trustee from the representative of my estate for any disbursement made by the Trustee pursuant hereto, nor shall there be any obligation upon such representative to repay to the Trustee any of the funds disbursed by it hereunder, and all amounts disbursed by the Trustee pursuant to the authority hereby conferred upon it shall be disbursed without any right in or duty upon the Trustee to seek or obtain contribution or reimbursement from any person or property on account of such payment. The Trustee shall not be responsible for the application of any funds delivered by it to the representative of my estate pursuant to the authority herein granted, nor shall the Trustee be subject to liability to any beneficiary hereunder on account of any payment made by it pursuant to the provisions hereof.

D. The Trustee shall keep accurate records showing all receipts and disbursements and other transactions involving the trust estate or estates and shall furnish annually to each beneficiary currently entitled to income, (1) a statement of the receipts and disbursements affecting such beneficiary's interest in the trust, and (2) a complete inventory of the trust estate then held for the benefit of such beneficiary.

E. No person, firm or corporation dealing with the Trustee or a nominee of the Trustee or performing any act pursuant to action taken or order given by the Trustee or such nominee shall be obliged to inquire as to the propriety, validity or legality thereof hereunder, nor shall any such person be liable for the application of any money or other consideration paid to the Trustee or such nominee, but, instead, may rely upon any action taken by the Trustee or such nominee pursuant to the powers and authorities conferred upon it under the provisions of this Article V in all respects as if the same were completely unlimited. No transfer agent or registrar of any security held hereunder shall be required to inquire as to the propriety, validity or legality of any transfer made by the Trustee or such nominee.

F. 1. In the event that said _____ shall be unwilling or unable to continue to serve as Trustee hereunder, then, my _____, _____, of _____, _____, shall serve as successor Trustee hereunder. In the event that both said _____ and said _____ shall be unwilling or unable to serve or continue to serve as Trustee hereunder, then _____, of _____, _____, shall serve as successor Trustee hereunder. Any Trustee shall be entitled to resign as Trustee for any reason whatsoever by giving written notice to the Trustee designated to succeed it; provided that the Trustee designated to succeed it shall first execute a formal written acceptance of the duties and obligations of the Trustee hereunder and file an executed copy of such acceptance with the preceding Trustee. After this is done, and when all sums then due from the trust estate to such predecessor Trustee have been paid, such predecessor Trustee shall transfer the Trust property then in its hands to such successor Trustee and such predecessor Trustee shall thereupon and thereby be discharged of all subsequent duties and obligations under or arising out of its trusteeship.

2. Any successor Trustee shall have and enjoy all the powers, authorities, duties and immunities hereby vested in and imposed upon the original Trustee and no successor Trustee shall be obliged to inquire into or be in any way accountable for the previous administration of the trust property.

G. My Trustee is authorized, in its discretion, to sell to, purchase from, borrow funds from, lend funds to, or otherwise deal with, upon such terms and conditions as my Trustee shall deem just and equitable and for full and adequate consideration, the Executor of the Last Will and Testament of myself or the Trustee of any Trust established by me (whether such Trust is a testamentary or inter vivos trust), even though my Trustee may also be serving as Executor under my Will or as Trustee under any such Trust established by me.

H. In determining the amount of any discretionary distributions of income or principal to a beneficiary of a trust created hereunder, the Trustee shall be required to take into account all other means and resources known to or reasonably ascertainable by the Trustee, including Medicaid or any other form of government assistance, which are available to such beneficiary for the purposes for which the Trustee is authorized to make said distributions.

I. _____, as Trustee, shall serve without compensation. Any other Trustee shall be entitled to receive reasonable compensation. Any Trustee shall be entitled to be reimbursed for reasonable expenses it incurs which are necessary to carry out its duties as Trustee hereunder.

J. No bond shall be required of the Trustee hereunder or any successor Trustee.

K. The Trustee and any successor Trustee are specifically instructed by the Settlor to maintain the privacy and confidentiality of this instrument and the trust created hereunder, and are in no circumstances to divulge its terms to any probate or other court or other public agency with the exception of a tax authority.

L. The Trustee and any successor Trustee shall have the authority to merge any trust held hereunder with any other trust, however created, which has similar provisions, the same beneficiaries and the same Trustee.

M. Notwithstanding any other provision contained herein, an individual Trustee (a) shall have no incident of ownership or power with respect to any policy of insurance upon such Trustee's life, and (b) shall have no power or discretion with respect to the allocation or distribution of assets to the extent that such would discharge such Trustee's legal obligation to support any beneficiary, or directly or indirectly benefit such Trustee unless necessary to provide for such Trustee's support in reasonable comfort, health care or education at any level, considering such Trustee's other financial resources.

ARTICLE VI
GOVERNING LAW

This Trust Agreement shall be construed under and in accordance with the laws of the State of _____.

IN WITNESS WHEREOF, I have hereunto set my hand, and the Trustee, to evidence its acceptance of the Trust herein expressed, has hereunto set its hand, in duplicate, at _____ _____, _____, on the day and year first above written.

Signed in the presence of:

_____   _____

_____   _____
                                                          "Settlor"

_____   _____

_____   _____
                                                          "Trustee"

STATE OF _____   City
                                       or
COUNTY OF _____   Town _____

    On the _____ day of _____, 19___, personally appeared
_____ known to me to be the individual(s) who executed the foregoing instrument, and acknowledged the same to be **[his/her]** free act and deed, before me.

_____
Notary Public

My commission expires:
_____

SCHEDULE A

The following is a true and correct Schedule A of the property assigned, delivered and conveyed to _____, Trustee, to be held, treated and disposed of in accordance with the terms of a certain Irrevocable Trust Agreement between _____, the Settlor, and _____, the Trustee, dated _____ ___, 19___, to which Agreement this Schedule A is attached and made a part thereof.

_____

_____

_____

_____

Signed in the presence of:

_____   _____

_____   _____

"Settlor"

_____   _____

_____   _____

"Trustee"

ADDITION OF PROPERTY TO IRREVOCABLE TRUST AGREEMENT

BY _____

DATED _____ ___, 19___

WITH _____, TRUSTEE

_____ (the "Assignor"), pursuant to the terms of the above-described Irrevocable Trust Agreement, does hereby assign, transfer and convey to _____,

Trustee, and _____

_____, Trustee, does hereby acknowledge receipt of, the following assets from the Assignor:

_____

_____

_____

_____

_____

_____

_____

_____

_____

_____

_____

_____

_____

_____

_____

_____

The Trustee agrees to hold, manage and administer the above assets as a part of the trust estate created under such Irrevocable Trust Agreement.

At the request of the Trustee, the Assignor shall fully cooperate and execute any and all documents deemed necessary or desirable by it in order to cause the assignment made hereby to be properly recorded.

IN WITNESS WHEREOF, the Assignor and the Trustee have signed their names at _____, _____, on this ____ day of _____, 19___.

Signed in the presence of:

_____

_____

_____

_____, Assignor

_____

_____, Trustee

STATE OF _____ City
or
COUNTY OF _____ Town _____

On the _____ day of _____, 19___, personally appeared
_____ known to me to be the individual(s) who executed the fore-
going instrument, and acknowledged the same to be **[his/her]** free act and deed, before me.

_____
Notary Public

My commission expires:

_____

Medicaid Trust No. 5
for Individual Who Is Unmarried, Leaving Assets to Children (Unequally) and/or to Others

Instructions/Explanation

As you can readily see, the trust agreement is filled with legalese. Don't be scared off by this confusing language. The explanations that follow should provide you with a clear understanding of the terms used.

Introduction: In the first blanks, fill in the city and state where you reside and the day, month, and year in which you are executing the Agreement.

Next, put in your name and residence (city and state)—the "Settlor" is your title when you make a trust. Then fill in the name, city, and state of the person or institution whom you are naming as trustee.

Remember, you should not be the trustee. A child or other close relative will probably be your first choice (keeping in mind possible tax consequences where annual distributions of over $10,000 will be made). If no one fits that description, you may have to name an institutional trustee, such as a bank.

Article I(A): This is the section making your trust irrevocable. Once you sign the Agreement, you will never be able to change, amend, or revoke it.

Article I(B): This paragraph transfers into the Trust all the items listed on Schedule A at the end of the Agreement. You can include on Schedule A just about any item imaginable, including real estate, personal property, savings and checking accounts, boats, cars, even clothing.

If the property you put into the trust increases in value, the increased value is part of the trust. And if an asset changes form, the new asset still remains in the trust. For example, if the trustee takes $5,000 from a bank account and buys $5,000 worth of stock, the stock remains in the trust.

While you can never remove assets once they are placed into the trust, you can always add to the trust by using the Addition to Trust form following Schedule A.

A testamentary gift, referred to in this paragraph, is a gift given at the time of someone's death, normally contained in a will. For example, you may not put your car into trust immediately, but you may add to your trust under your will when you die.

Article II: This section gives you the income from the trust during your life, but specifically provides that you cannot get at the principal. This is *absolutely crucial* to saving your estate from the grasp of a nursing home if you enter one. With this language, Medicaid cannot require you to spend the principal on the nursing home *because you don't control or even have access to the principal.*

Why does the Trust Agreement give discretion to the Trustee to pay you income rather than *requiring* the Trustee to pay you all the income? Because with this provision, you *may* be able to protect your income from the nursing home.

Let's say the Trust Agreement just said that all the income was automatically yours. If you entered a nursing home, Medicaid would force you to pay all the income to the nursing home and would only cover any deficiency on the bill. But if the Trustee has discretion to decide whether or not to pay all the income to you, after you go into a nursing home the Trustee might decide *not* to pay *any* of the income to you. In that situation, Medicaid might pay the entire nursing-home tab, because you don't have any income. (I say might because the law and its application to situations like this are not yet clear. It is possible that Medicaid might say that, even if you're not actually receiving any income, you *could* receive some or all of the income and so it won't pay the full nursing-home bill.)

Article III: This section describes how your trust principal, less any of your estate taxes, estate administration costs, or funeral expenses as provided in Article V(C), will be distributed after you die.

Paragraph III(A) provides that, after you die, the balance of your trust principal will be distributed to the persons you list in the Trust in the proportions you set. You can name anyone you choose: children, other family members, friends. You can also fix whatever percentages you wish; just make sure the percentages add up exactly to 100%. If any person named in the trust has died before you, that person's portion goes to his or her children. A trust alternatively could provide that a deceased's beneficiary's portion would be divided among the then-living named beneficiaries; if you'd prefer that arrangement, have your lawyer revise this section.

Paragraph III(B) provides for the distribution of the trust if there's no one to receive the principal from your trust under Paragraph III(A).

Under III(B), the remaining principal of the trust will be divided into two parts. One part will go to those persons who would inherit from you under the laws of your state as if you had died without a will or a trust. Every state has a law that dictates to whom an estate of someone who dies without a will will be distributed—usually to the closest living relative(s) of the deceased. For example, if you die without children or grandchildren, Paragraph III(B) may mean that your parent or brother collects part of the trust estate.

The other half of the trust estate will be distributed to those persons who would inherit from your deceased spouse under the laws of your state as if he or she had died without a will.

The estate is split into two parts so that relatives on both sides of your family are treated equally. For example, rather than having everything go to your cousin, half may go to your cousin and half to your deceased spouse's sister.

Fill in the blanks in Paragraph III(B) with the names of your state and your deceased spouse (if any).

Part III(C) discusses distributions, after you die, to beneficiaries named in your trust who are under some legal disability or are unable to administer their distributions. For example, if your child is to receive a distribution and he or she is senile or suffering from Alzheimer's disease, he or she may be under a legal disability or unable to manage his or her money. Or if a distribution under your trust is to go to a young child (perhaps the children of a deceased child of yours), Part III(C) may come into play.

If a distribution from your trust is to go to someone who is under a legal disability or unable to manage their money, the Trustee has four options:

1. Pay the money to the beneficiary.
2. Make the distribution to a legal guardian of the beneficiary.
3. Distribute the beneficiary's portion to a custodian for the beneficiary.
4. Spend the money himself or herself for the benefit of the beneficiary.

If, when you make up your trust, you could predict the ages and physical and mental conditions of all your beneficiaries at the time of your death, you could spell out which of these four options you would want the Trustee to pursue. But since you can't, this Trust allows the Trustee to choose which option he or she believes is best.

The last sentence of Part III(C) says that, once the Trustee has made his or her choice and distributed a beneficiary's portion to the beneficiary or to the beneficiary's guardian or custodian, the Trustee is off the hook; he or she doesn't have to monitor the use of the distribution after that.

Part III(D), often called a spendthrift clause, provides that nobody but your intended beneficiary can obtain an interest in a distribution under your Trust. For example, your child, who will receive a portion of your Trust after you're gone, can't sell his or her expected distribution in the future to someone for cash now. And a beneficiary can't put up his or her interest in a distribution as collateral for a loan. After all, you want the person you name in the Trust to receive a distribution, not some stranger.

Spendthrift clauses like this are enforced in most, but not all, states. If you have a serious concern that a beneficiary has or may have creditor problems, consult with a local attorney to determine whether this clause will be effective in your state.

Trusts cannot legally tie up assets forever, so Part III(E) is designed to avoid potential problems by limiting the life of the Trust.

Article IV: This is the definition section. The only important point here is to recognize that a legally adopted child will be considered a child for purposes of the Trust Agreement.

Article V: This section deals with the powers and duties you are giving to the Trustee.

Part V(A) says that, after your death, the Trustee must collect the money due under any insurance policy on your life. The Trustee does not have a duty to pay your life insurance premiums during your lifetime, until and unless the Trustee takes title to any insurance policy.

Part V(B) is very important, setting forth the powers of the Trustee. As you can see, this Trust Agreement gives the Trustee very broad powers to administer the funds and property in the estate, including the power to:

1. Buy real estate or personal property from your estate. Without this power, purchases by your Trustee from your estate at death might not be allowed.
2. Keep in the Trust anything received from you or your estate.
3. Sell, exchange, mortgage, and do just about anything else with property in the Trust.
4. Invest the assets in the Trust in just about anything.
5. Borrow money for the Trust.
6. Manage stock and other securities.
7. Collect money for the Trust.
8. Handle claims and lawsuits for or against the Trust.
9. Hire and pay counselors and assistants, like lawyers and accountants, for the Trust.
10. Hold property in his or her own name, in the name of a nominee, or in bearer form.
11. Manage real estate in the Trust, including repairing, improving, or converting property.
12. Handle life insurance policies in the Trust, including paying premiums, canceling or selling policies, cashing in policies, or borrowing against them.
13. Make distributions under the Trust in cash or in property.
14. Receive additional property for the Trust.
15. Do anything else reasonably required to manage, protect, or preserve the Trust assets.

Why put in many specific powers, instead of just having item 15, which generally allows the Trustee to do anything reasonably necessary? Because with only a general statement, someone with whom the Trustee must deal may question his or her power and may refuse to do business with him or her. For example, without specifically giving the Trustee the power to sell real estate, buyers, lenders, and escrow agents may be hesitant to deal with him or her, even if your trust agreement generally gives him or her broad powers. By listing specific powers, you can ensure the Trustee's ability properly to manage the Trust.

Why give the Trustee such broad powers anyway? Why not just specify a few actions he or she may take? The reason is simple: you can't predict what the Trustee may need to do to manage your estate properly, and if you don't give him or her broad powers, you may hamper him or her and damage your Trust estate. For example, if you don't own any stocks, why give the Trustee power to manage them? Because at some point it might be in your best interest for your Trustee to purchase securities, and your Trust Agreement could unnecessarily prevent him or her from doing so.

Part V(C) provides for certain payments from your Trust upon your death. If the representative of your estate (such as the executor or administrator) decides that the funds left in your estate (not in your Trust) are insufficient to pay your estate taxes, expenses of administration, or funeral expenses, he or she can require the Trustee to cover those costs. The Trustee does not have to get anything in return, and your estate representative does not have to repay the money. Once the Trustee has paid the representative of your estate, the Trustee has no further obligation to monitor the use of these funds.

Part V(D) requires the Trustee to keep accurate records showing all transactions in the Trust. Every year, the Trustee must give to certain beneficiaries a statement listing the Trust transactions for the year and a current inventory of assets in the Trust. Not every possible future beneficiary of the Trust gets this report. For example, if the Trust Agreement provides income to you for your lifetime, then on your death the assets will be distributed to your children or their children, only you are entitled to the Trustee's report.

Part V(E) is designed to encourage people to deal with the Trustee by relieving them of liability in case the Trustee takes some action beyond his power. For example, if the Trustee attempts to sell a house, the buyer can go ahead with the transaction and pay the Trustee without worrying about whether the Trust really allows the Trustee to make that deal.

Part V(F)(1) allows you to name alternative Trustees in case your first and/or second choice can't or won't serve when the time comes. In the first blank, put the name of your first choice for Trustee. In the next three blanks, fill in the relationship to you, the name and residence of your second choice. In the next two blanks, fill in the names of your first and second choices for Trustee. In the last three blanks, include the name, city, and state of a third choice for Trustee.

Part V(F)(2) gives any successor Trustee all the

same powers and duties as the original Trustee. It also encourages your chosen successor Trustee to accept the job by providing that he or she has no responsibility for anything done by the earlier Trustee.

Part V(G) authorizes the Trustee to engage in transactions with the Executor of your estate or any trustee of any other trust established by you. Without this language, a conflict-of-interest issue could arise over these types of dealings.

Part V(H) concerns discretionary distributions by the Trustee. Under Article II, the Trustee is given discretion to distribute to you all the net income of the trust. Let's say you enter a nursing home—will some or all of the income from the trust have to be paid to the nursing home? Under the law as it stands now, the answer is not totally clear. Medicaid may take the position that *all* the income must be paid to you (and so to the nursing home). But with Part V(H), there is a chance you can save part or all of the income.

Under Part V(H), the Trustee could decide not to pay any of the income to you. In fact, by requiring the Trustee to consider other resources available, including Medicaid, you are tilting the Trustee's decision in the direction of nonpayment. If the Trustee makes that decision, Medicaid might allow the trust to retain the income while it pays your nursing-home costs.

In Part V(I), you are providing that the Trustee (whose name must be filled in the blank) will serve without compensation. Since the Trustee will probably be your child or someone else close to you, that should be agreeable. Other possible trustees, such as a bank, will want to be paid, and Part V(I) allows that as well.

Part V(J) states that the Trustee does not have to post a bond. A bond is like an insurance policy, designed to protect your Trust in case the Trustee does something wrong, such as steals assets. Depending on the amount in the Trust, the bond could easily cost your Trust several hundred dollars. If you've followed the tips in this book and selected the right Trustee, you shouldn't need a bond.

Part V(K) instructs the Trustee to keep the terms of your Trust private to the maximum extent possible. A trust has a great advantage over a will when it comes to passing your assets along after your death. Your estate becomes an open book when it goes through probate; when it passes under a trust, it can be kept from the eyes of nosy neighbors.

Part V(L) allows the Trustee to merge trusts that are very similar to avoid duplication of effort and costs.

Part V(M) is a protection for the Trustee to avoid the remote possibility of having the trust property included in the Trustee's estate, causing adverse tax consequences.

Article VI: Article VI states that any questions about the Trust will be answered by the laws of the state of your primary residence. In the blank space, fill in the name of your state.

Conclusion: In the blanks in the final paragraph, fill in your city and state. Then sign where it says Settlor (that's you) and have the Trustee sign below that. You and the Trustee should each print your names below the signature lines. To the left of your and the Trustee's signatures, two witnesses to each signature must sign. The witnesses can be the same, but they don't have to be; if they are the same, they must sign twice (once for the Settlor and once for the Trustee). The witnesses cannot be members of your family.

The final section is for a notary public.

Schedule A: Following the end of the Trust is Schedule A, on which you should list any items (i.e., cash accounts, real estate, personal property, etc.) to be placed under the control of the Trustee. Identify each item as best you can, using addresses, registration numbers, account numbers, etc., wherever possible, to avoid confusion.

On Schedule A, fill in: the name of the Trustee in the first blank, your name (the "Settlor") in the second blank, and the name of the Trustee again in the third blank. Then date the Schedule.

At the bottom, you and the Trustee should sign before two independent witnesses.

Addition of Property Form: Finally included is a form that you can use to add property to the Trust later. At the top, fill in your name, the date that the Trust was originally made, and the name of the Trustee. In the first full paragraph, fill in your name as the Assignor, assigning property to the Trustee. Then on the lines that follow, list any items to be added to the Trust. Again, identify each item as best you can. At the end, you and the Trustee should sign before two independent witnesses and a notary.

Notes

Introduction

1. Statement of Representative Claude M. Pepper, "Catastrophic Health Insurance: Filling the Long-Term Care Gap," Hearing before the Subcommittee on Health and Long-Term Care of the House of Representatives Select Committee on Aging, July 2, 1987 ("July 2 Hearing"), p. 5.

2. Statement of Jack Ossofsky, "Paying the Price of Catastrophic Illness: From Accidents to Alzheimer's," Hearing before the Subcommittee on Health and Long-Term Care of the House of Representatives Select Committee on Aging, January 28, 1987 ("January 28 Hearing"), p. 29.

3. Statement of Grace Still, "Catastrophic Health Insurance: The Pennsylvania Perspective," Hearing before the Subcommittee on Health and Long-Term Care of the House of Representatives Select Committee on Aging, April 10, 1987 ("April 10 Hearing"), pp. 13–14.

4. Statement of Nathan Mendelsohn, April 10 Hearing, pp. 12–13.

5. Statement of Representative Robert A. Borski, April 10 Hearing, p. 3.

6. Statement of Esther Peterson, United Press International, article by Ken Franckling, December 7, 1987.

7. Statement of Senator John Heinz, Associated Press, article by Margaret Scherf, September 21, 1984.

Chapter 1

1. Figures from the U.S. Department of Health and Human Services, set forth in "Long Term Care and Personal Impoverishment: Seven in Ten Elderly Living Alone Are at Risk," report presented by the Chairman of the Select Committee on Aging of the House of Representatives, October 1987, p. 5.

2. Esther Peterson, *Choice Time: Thinking Ahead on Long Term Care*, prepared by Aetna Life Insurance and Annuity Company, undated.

3. Statement of Representative Mary Rose Oakar, Hearing before the Subcommittee on Health and Long-Term Care of the House of Representatives Select Committee on Aging, July 2, 1987 ("July 2 Hearing"), p. 16.

4. Statement of Representative Edward R. Roybal, news release of the House of Representatives Select Committee on Aging, November 9, 1987.

5. Letter of Mrs. Bellamy, Knoxville, Tennessee, presented in Statement of William A. Lessard, July 2 Hearing, p. 84.

6. Attachment to Testimony of Dr. Samuel L. Baily, Hearing before the Subcommittee on Health and Long-Term Care of the House of Representatives Select Committee on Aging, January 28, 1987 ("January 28 Hearing"), p. 156.

7. Testimony of Dr. Samuel L. Baily, January 28 Hearing, p. 136.

8. Statement of Representative Claude M. Pepper, "Catastrophic Health Insurance: The Pennsylvania Perspective," Hearing before the Subcommittee on Health and Long-Term Care of the House of Representatives Select Committee on Aging, April 10, 1987, p. 15.

Chapter 2

1. Statement of Representative Robert A. Borski, "Catastrophic Health Insurance: The Pennsylvania Perspective," Hearing before the Subcommittee on Health and Long-Term Care of the House of Representatives Select Committee on Aging, April 10, 1987 ("April 10 Hearing"), p. 15.

2. Statement of Jack J. Lomas, April 10 Hearing, p. 10.

3. Statement of Representative Robert A. Borski, April 10 Hearing, p. 3.

4. Statement of Representative Claude Pepper, April 10 Hearing, p. 8.

5. Statement of Gail Shearer, Hearing before the Subcommittee on Health and Long-Term Care of the House of Representatives Select Committee on Aging, January 28, 1987 ("January 28 Hearing"), p. 53.

6. Statement of Gail Shearer, January 28 Hearing, p. 57.

7. Statement of Val J. Halamandaris, January 28 Hearing, p. 50.

8. From Statement of William A. Lessard, Hearing before the Subcommittee on Health and Long-Term Care of the House of Representatives Select Committee on Aging, July 2, 1987, p. 84.

9. "Long Term Care and Personal Impoverishment: Seven in Ten Elderly Living Alone Are at Risk," Report presented by the Chairman of the Select Committee on Aging of the House of Representatives, October 1987, p. 3.

Acknowledgments

This book would not have been possible without the help, support, and understanding of a lot of people.

First, I would like to thank my wife, Amy. Amy should actually be listed as a co-author, given the number of hours she spent working on the manuscript. Amy is my partner, my inspiration—and my number-one editor.

Very special thanks to Patricia Nemore, staff attorney for the National Senior Citizens Law Center, who knows more about the Medicare Catastrophic Coverage Act than anyone else in the country, and Michael Schuster, director of litigation for the Legal Counsel for the Elderly. Trish and Mike spent many, many hours working with me to make sure the book is accurate. Their help has been absolutely invaluable.

In the book are frequent references to a report prepared by Edward Neuschler for the National Governors' Association. That report contains a wealth of information, and I appreciate Mr. Neuschler's and the National Governors' Association's permission to provide portions of it to you.

Thanks also to Laura B. Wallens and Frank C. Krasovec, Jr., attorneys in my office, who helped prepare many of the forms; the management of my law firm, Hahn Loeser & Parks, which has always supported my public-service efforts; Esther Peterson, Edith Furst, and my agent, Barbara Lowenstein, whose guidance helped shape the proper approach; and David Guralnik, whose support encouraged me to pursue this effort.

I can't omit Arthur Hettich. Arthur had the wisdom to give me my first "big break" by accepting my articles for *Family Circle* magazine. I would also like to thank Ellen Stoianoff, my editor at *Family Circle*, and my editors at the *Cleveland Plain Dealer*, who helped teach me how to write clearly for non-lawyers.

I must thank Congressman Claude Pepper and his staff for their enthusiastic support and persistent advocacy on behalf of older Americans.

Finally, thanks to my kids, Ryan and Daniel, who hopefully won't have to worry about me in my old age, and to my parents, for whom I wish a long and healthy life—I love you all.